PROBLEMS OF APHASIA

NEUROLINGUISTICS

An International Series Devoted to Speech Physiology
and Speech Pathology

Edited by

Richard Hoops, Ph.D. and *Yvan Lebrun*, Ph.D.

1979

SWETS & ZEITLINGER B. V. – LISSE

PROBLEMS
OF APHASIA

Edited by

Yvan Lebrun and *Richard Hoops*

1979

SWETS & ZEITLINGER B. V. – LISSE

Set by Western Printing Services Limited, Bristol, England
Printed in Holland by Offsetdrukkerij Kanters B.V., Alblasserdam

ISBN 90 265 0309 1

CONTENTS

CONTRIBUTORS

SUE ANDERSON DAVIS, Speech, Language and Hearing Clinic, Ball State University, Muncie, Indiana 47306 (U.S.A.).

RICHARD ARTES, Ph.D., Speech, Language and Hearing Clinic, Ball State University, Muncie, Indiana 47306 (U.S.A.).

GILBERT ASSAL, M.D., Service de Neurochirurgie, Centre Hospitalier Universitaire Vaudois, 1011 Lausanne (Switzerland).

FRANÇOIS BOLLER, M.D., Department of Neurology, University of Pittsburgh School of Medicine, 322 Scaife Hall, Pittsburgh, PA 15261, U.S.A.

JOCELYNE BUTTET, Service de Neurochirurgie, Centre Hospitalier Universitaire Vaudois, 1011 Lausanne (Switzerland).

ANDRÉA COLLIER, M.D., Département de Neurologie, Hôpital d'Ixelles, 63 rue Jean Paquot, 1050 Bruxelles (Belgium).

RICHARD HOOPS, Ph.D., Speech, Language and Hearing Clinic, Ball State University, Muncie, Indiana 47306 (U.S.A.).

GUDRUN KAISER, Neurolinguïstiek, Consultatiegebouw, Akademisch Ziekenhuis V.U.B., Laarbeeklaan, 1090 Brussel (Belgium).

YVAN LEBRUN, Ph.D., Neurolinguïstiek, Consultatiegebouw, Akademisch Ziekenhuis V.U.B., Laarbeeklaan, 1090 Brussel (Belgium).

CHANTAL LELEUX, Clinique Neurochirurgicale, Université Libre de Bruxelles, 1 rue Héger-Bordet, 1000 Bruxelles (Belgium).

KARL LEONHARD, M.D., Bereich Medizin (Charité), Nervenklinik, Schumannstrasse 20/21, 104 Berlin (German Democratic Republic).

GUY MONSEU, M.D., Département de Neurologie, Hôpital de Saint-Gilles, rue Marconi, 1180 Bruxelles (Belgium).

NICOLAS STOUPEL, M.D., Département de Neurologie, Hôpital d'Ixelles, 63 rue Jean Paquot, 1050 Bruxelles (Belgium).

ERIC ZANDER, M.D., Service de Neurochirurgie, Centre Hospitalier Universitaire Vaudois, 1011 Lausanne (Switzerland).

INTRODUCTION

The present volume comprises three parts.

The first part, which includes four papers, addresses itself to the pathology of the dominant hemisphere. The first two contributions deal with aphasic disorders and with alexic disturbances resulting from a retro-rolandic lesion. The third paper compares the verbal behaviours of various types of aphasics under circumstances of delayed auditory feedback, while the fourth presentation examines whether in aphasics verbal expression and pantomime abilities are equally impaired.

The second part, which comprises two papers, focusses on the pathology of the minor hemisphere. One of the papers studies voice identification by right brain damaged patients as compared with normals and left brain damaged subjects. The second contribution reports a case of dyscalculia due to a lesion of the minor hemisphere.

The last paper, finally, approaches the problem of linguistic attainments of subjects who have had to undergo the resection of one cerebral hemisphere.

1

IDEOKINETIC APHASIA AND RELATED DISORDERS

KARL LEONHARD

When undertaking to describe a special form of aphasia and its special localization justification is necessary; for many, today, refuse to believe that there are different aphasias which can be differently localized. The doctrines of Broca, Wernicke, Liepmann, Dejerine, and Lichtheim are completely rejected by some aphasiologists, who maintain that neurophysiological investigations as well as linguistic research have demonstrated that the structure and function of normal language must be taken much more into consideration than the classical authors did. Assal (1965) is of the opinion that as regards the controversy between Pierre Marie and Dejerine most French authors today follow Marie. In German literature Bay has repeatedly contradicted the classical views and defended the conceptions of Pierre Marie. In Bay's opinion, aphasia is a disturbance of conceptional thinking, which implies that one cannot distinguish various types of aphasia. Most authors do not agree with this view, as could be seen at an international conference on intelligence and aphasia, in Brussels a few years ago. At this conference (Lebrun and Hoops, 1974) Bay recalled his well-known observations that clay models and drawings, made from memory by aphasics, are defective. Leischner contradicted this assertion. In his clinic occupational therapy includes drawing, painting, and clay modeling. Impairment could only be found in those patients who in addition to aphasia had a parietal syndrome with constructional difficulties. Poeck agreed with Leischner, confirming that some drawings and clay models in Leischner's collections were really artistic, although made by patients with severe aphasia. Goodglass maintained that aphasics have intellectual deficits in recovering and using the elements which make up a total concept, but they appear to be free from impairment in the logical approach

11

to problem solving. He mentioned a patient who in spite of severe aphasia and a complete agraphia attained a performance IQ of 112 on the Wechsler Adult Intelligence Scale. Welman and Lanser reported the case of a 50 year old female with a very severe motor aphasia, who could make herself understood only by intonation and gestures. Nonetheless, she was able to perform her work as a house-wife and to do shopping correctly. Zangwill quoted Pierre Marie's opinion that occupational competence is necessarily affected in aphasia and discussed the aphasic patient of Marie who, though being a professional chef, failed to produce a dish of fried eggs upon request. Zangwill contrasted to this patient another aphasic man, whose speech was virtually nonexistent and who had yet been working quite successfully for a number of years as an assistant chef and discharged his duties to the complete satisfaction of his superiors. Messerli and Tissot maintained that the classification tests they used did not confirm Bay's theory: aphasics found these tests difficult because they required verbal mediation. The two authors also referred to the examination of 218 patients performed by Tissot, Lhermitte and Ducarne (1963). Some of these patients, though severely aphasic, showed no intellectual reduction in non-verbal tests.

It appears, therefore, that aphasia is a specific disorder. Of course intelligence must be affected when inner speech, which so facilitates thinking, is disturbed. It would be very astonishing if it were not so. The fact that we can find severe disorders of speaking combined with only slight disorders of thinking in itself demonstrates that language and thought are two different functions.

It is another question whether there is only one aphasic entity, or whether there are several aphasic forms which must be distinguished. Today many authors no longer separate different forms because there are so many mixed cases. But really, this is not decisive, since we cannot expect lesions in the brain to be limited to areas united in function. On the other hand, the number of mixed cases significantly diminishes if one takes into account ideokinetic aphasia, which is so frequently considered mixed motor and sensory aphasia since there are not only articulatory difficulties but also paraphasias. If one takes ideokinetic aphasia into consideration one in fact observes many more pure cases than Leischner, who in a group of 400 cases found only 23 pure motor aphasias, 6 pure sensory aphasias and 7 pure amnestic aphasias (Lebrun and Hoops, 1974, p. 99). Actually ideokinetic aphasia is not more rare than sensory aphasia, and occurs much more frequently than cortical dysarthria. Because ideokinetic aphasia is neglected, disagreements are mostly about the disturbances of expressive speech. Bay (1957) rightly maintains that motor aphasia as conceived of by Broca and localized in the third frontal convolution, does not exist. Lesions of this region produce speech disorders which really are better termed dysarthria than aphasia. But this does not mean that independent motor aphasias do not exist at all. We shall speak about this later.

Regarding localization of disorders in the brain, modern views, in spite of Bay's objections, are more related to the classical doctrine of regions and neural connections. Disconnection syndromes are being discussed again with great interest, since Geschwind (1965) and others re-directed attention to them. Lhermitte and Beauvois (1973) expressed the opinion that these syndromes have been too much neglected. However, when Leonhard in 1952 (a) described pure agraphia and constructional apraxia in consequence of disconnection, Conrad (1953) purposely published an article which was to demonstrate that according to modern knowledge it was no longer justifiable to derive psychological disorders from disconnection.

Where there are connections, there must be regions being connected. Regarding the alleged brain centres, modern views are certainly quite different from the classical opinions. But also in the neurological sphere we can no longer speak of centers as earlier authors did. The statement that certain regions are of special significance for neuropsychological functions, especially for language, is not contradicted. Lhermitte and Gautier (1969) write: 'Cerebral regions, damage of which causes aphasia, are obviously necessary pieces in the mechanisms of speech but they are no more "language centres" than the precentral gyrus is the centre of movement.' Some modern authors even think that intelligence also is anatomically based in certain regions of the brain. Poeck (in Lebrun and Hoops, 1974, p. 126) agrees on this point with Basso, De Renzi, Faglioni, Scotti and Spinnler (1973). It would seem, however, that only the means of mental activity (cp. 'Werkzeugstörungen' in Lange, 1936) are connected with certain regions, whereas intelligence appears to have its basis in all parts of the hemisphere.

The temporary rejection of disconnection syndromes as introduced by the classical authors resulted from the rejection of associative psychology. Still, there is an important difference. Associative psychologists were of the opinion that they could, referring to associations, explain the totality of psychic events, whereas Wernicke, Dejerine, Liepmann and others only wanted to explain some performances of mental activity. Since the hemispheres for the greater part consist of associative fibers, it would be highly astonishing if connections were not of eminent importance. In practice it is confirmed that there are different regions of different functions connected with each other. The practical neurologist successfully relates neuro-psychological defects to certain regions of the brain. He will be even more successful if he knows the parietal form of aphasia.

1. *The nature of ideokinetic aphasia*

For many years neurologists have been aware of the relationship of motor aphasia to apraxia. Liepmann (1900), after having discovered apraxia, compared this disturbance with motor aphasia and explained in detail that in motor aphasia as well as in melokinetic ('gliedki-netisch') apraxia the kinetic memory was disturbed, i.e. the kinesthetic memory and at the same time the memory for the patterns of movements. In this view the term *kinesthetic* is of importance. Liepmann's theory, which was accepted by many authors, implies that melo-kinetic apraxia, which Kleist (1934) later called *innervatory apraxia*, is also based on disorders in the kinesthetic sphere. When Niessl von Mayendorf (1930) termed motor aphasia *amnesia verbalis kinaes-thetica*, he also indicated a relationship to melokinetic apraxia. In more recent times Nielsen (1946) took a similar view. Speaking of *apraxic aphasia* he likewise established a parallel with melokinetic apraxia. Ideokinetic apraxia is described by him, but is not discussed in relation to aphasia. Luria (1966), who connects a kinesthetic (parietal) form of aphasia with a kinesthetic (likewise parietal) form of apraxia, describes the breaks in speaking, which characterize ideokinetic aphasia, in regard to efferent motor aphasia and not in regard to kinesthetic aphasia. Konorski (1970), on the other hand, speaks of kinesthetic disorders in Broca's aphasia, again indicating localization in the frontal lobe, agreeing with former authors.

Liepmann had assumed ideokinetic apraxia to be produced by dissociation of the idea, aiming at movements, from the corresponding melokinetic patterns. Dejerine (1914) developed the same theory and spoke of apraxia of transmission. This opinion, even from the

14

classical point of view, can no longer be supported. Kleist (1934) derives ideokinetic apraxia from a loss of the kinesthetic engrams, and innervatory apraxia from a loss of the innervatory memory for complex movements. Instead of ideokinetic apraxia Kleist sometimes uses the term *kinesthetic apraxia*. Though Luria (1966) also speaks of kinesthetic apraxia, the two authors do not agree as to meaning. Kleist thinks of the loss of memory-images in the sense of the classical doctrine, while Luria supposes 'a disturbance in the ability to integrate single stimuli into simultaneous structures or groups'. An aphasia of this nature, characterized by a loss of memory-images (Kleist), or loss of ability to integrate (Luria), was described for the first time by Leonhard in 1954. To be sure, the idea of this type of aphasia occasionally arose before. In the examination of patients suffering from conduction aphasia (repetition aphasia) Kleist (1934) regularly found the supramarginal gyrus affected. He mentioned in this connection that the speech disorder in pronunciation often gave the impression of apraxia. And he added: 'It therefore might be possible that repetition aphasia includes an apraxic component.'

When defining an apraxic form of motor aphasia we have to focus upon the parietal lobe, since ideokinetic apraxia results from lesions of this lobe, especially of the supramarginal gyrus. The parietal lobe is often said to be of significance in speaking. Pötzl (1925), referring to several cases he had observed, speaks of parietal-linked aphasia and also mentions the clinical similarity to conduction aphasia. However, he does not presume a relationship to apraxia, but assumes that the inferior region of the parietal lobe subserves the organization of language. Niessl von Mayendorf (1930), however, denied that the parietal lobe was of significance for speaking.

As ideokinetic aphasia really presents a certain similarity to the syndrome described under the name of conduction aphasia or central aphasia, in which the repetition of spoken words is particularly and grossly impaired, it is interesting to note where lesions have been found in this latter form of aphasia. Goldstein (1914) admitted a lesion in the insular region: 'So the clinical syndrome corresponds to conduction aphasia rather well. And there is anatomically a lesion of that speech area in which resides, I suppose, the central speech apparatus (like Storch and Kleist), i.e. the insular region.' The lesion, however, was not confined to this region. Regarding the parietal lobe Goldstein noted: 'Supramarginal gyrus, cortex as well as subcortical and deep white matter, are extremely damaged; similarly angular gyrus and anterior part of the inferior parietal gyrus.' That such extensive destruction could be neglected was only possible because the parietal lobe was excluded from discussions about aphasia. This has not changed in our time. Russel and Espir (1961) could recognize the great significance of the parietal lobe in their 250 brain injured aphasic patients, for, according to their diagrams, the parietal lobe was much more frequently damaged than the frontal lobe and even the temporal lobe. Yet these authors do not attempt to derive a special form of aphasia from the lesions of the parietal lobe.

Sometimes, however, the idea arises that the disturbance of repetition, the principal symptom of conduction aphasia, results from damage to the parietal lobe. Shortly after publication of Leonhard's paper on kinetic aphasia (1954), Stengel and Patch (1955), reporting three cases of central aphasia associated with parietal symptoms, suggested replacing the term *central aphasia* with *temporo-parietal aphasia*. Benson and Geschwind (1969) in the *Handbook of Clinical Neurology* expressed the opinion that the lesion in conduction aphasia had an extension from the parietal operculum to the angular gyrus. In the middle of this extension lies the supramarginal gyrus which we regard as essentially affected. Benson and Geschwind also remarked that this type of aphasia is not rare. It is also important that Kohlmeyer (1970) considers conduction aphasia an almost specific syndrome of the posterior parietal artery and angular gyrus artery. He is furthermore of the opinion that occlusion of the latter usually produces a Gerstmann syndrome, whereas occlusion of the former usually produces conduction aphasia. So we are again directed to the supramarginal gyrus.

Motor aphasias are especially found associated with buccofacial apraxia. The relationship has been known since Jackson (1932) described this form of apraxia. In recent years such a relationship was assumed by Hartl (1964), De Renzi, Pieczuro and Vignolo (1966), Poggi (1968), Gimeno (1969), but the ideokinetic and the innervatory form of buccofacial apraxia are not sufficiently separated. Ajuriaguerra and Tissot (1969), in the *Handbook of Clinical Neurology*, describe only one buccofacial apraxia. We agree with these authors that innervatory apraxia is regularly associated with dysarthria. But the ideokinetic form has a different feature and is differently related to aphasia. A typical ideokinetic form of buccofacial apraxia was

16

described by Lhermitte in a discussion (see Leischner, 1970), but he related it to Wernicke's aphasia.

In limbs, innervatory apraxia is characterized by lack of skill and rapidity, without the movements being distorted. The finer the movement, the more difficult it is for the patient, so that the hand or the fingers often do not move at all for a moment. In ideokinetic apraxia the movements are not so labored, but there occur constant slips or derailments into wrong movements. In the same way the two forms of buccofacial apraxia differ from each other. In the innervatory form the movements of the eyes, cheeks, lips and tongue are not incorrectly carried out, but are performed slowly, laboriously, and somewhat crudely. Often they are only half finished or remain undone. During World War II Domnick (1943), a disciple of Kleist's, described several patients suffering from innervatory facial apraxia after gunshot injuries. Only his case No. 3 (Krau) is not typical because of his slips into wrong movements. These slips, also found in the facial form, are characteristic of ideokinetic apraxia. Innervatory apraxia has reference to cortical dysarthria, in which the speech movements are not incorrect but are crudely performed. They also are slow and labored, which is how cortical dysarthria differs from pseudobulbar dysarthria.

Let us now consider our own case material.

Case No. 1. Augusta Fel., born 1894, housewife. In the winter of 1950/51 she was struck with apoplexy, after which she could only mumble. There was a paralysis of the right arm. In the spring of 1951 the patient gradually recovered her speech faculty but remained unable to formulate complete sentences. The paralysis of the arm improved. The patient was not admitted to a hospital but was attended by a neighbour living on the same floor. In June she was very much alarmed because her son was sent to prison. After that, she spoke very little, barricaded the door, listened constantly to detect whether her son might not be coming. In June, 1951 she was admitted to the University Clinic in Frankfurt/Main, where she stayed for six weeks.

Fel. was sad and complained of her son having been taken away. By diverting her attention, it was possible to appease and to cheer her up.

In this pyknic and slightly obese woman a blood-pressure of 210/

17

120 was found. The right arm was still paretic but could be moved, and the legs were not paretic. There was no definite paresis of the facial nerve. Tendon and periosteal reflexes were all brisk on the right side; Babinski's sign was positive. Sensibility was somewhat dulled on the entire right side. There was a homonymous narrowing of the right side of the visual field. In addition there were difficulties in distinguishing between right and left and in recognizing fingers, as well as constructional apraxia. The patient also read very incorrectly, a disturbance to which the difficulties in pronunciation contributed. Some written words could not be understood. There was a severe writing disorder, most letters being distorted and some being unrecognizable. Copying was less disturbed, but some letters were deformed. With the left hand the patient wrote even more incorrectly. There was acalculia, but it was difficult to decide how far the speech and writing disorders accounted for it. Orientation as to place was good, but orientation as to time was not. The patient could not indicate the year, month, or day of the week. This defect was not due to disturbance of memory, for the patient was always well aware of the events in her surroundings and could remember when she had been visited, who had come to see her, when and how often she had been examined. The general behaviour of the patient was normal; she also had insight into her illness.

The following findings are given in detail because they demonstrate the special features of ideokinetic apraxia and ideokinetic aphasia.

APRAXIA OF THE HANDS. *Beckoning right hand*: Correct, but clumsy. *Left hand*: The same, but in addition unnecessary movements of the fingers. *Thumbing her nose*: Holds her left hand in front of her face. When shown how to do it, she directs the forefinger to her nose. *Right hand*: She holds the hand as a fist near the nose. *Threatening*: She simply lifts her right hand as well as her left hand. When shown how to do it with the forefinger, with the left she shakes her hand forward and backward. On the right she gradually succeeds regarding the posture of the finger, but now lifts her hand without moving it. After being shown several times how to do it, she succeeds once, but only transiently; then she again holds the fingers in a wrong way. In repetition of the trial on the left side, she first lifts only her hand, then suddenly she succeeds perfectly. *Turning a coffee grinder*: She describes a circle on the table-top, on the right as well as on the left, without the hands having the correct posture. *Saluting*: She holds

18

the hand as a fist near the cheek, then tries a little and now holds the flat hand near the cheek. Spontaneously she adds the left hand and now holds both her hands near the cheeks. *Turning on the water-tap*: She moves her hand like turning a coffee mill, though she was unable to produce this very movement a little earlier. On the left she first tries a little, then moves her hand in the same way as she did on the right.

There are her movements on command and by imitation. In real situations, handling actual objects, the patient acts correctly. She cannot make the gesture of knocking when she has nothing to knock at, but with either hand, she adequately knocks at a folder which is held in front of her and represents a door. She is perfectly successful in handling a candle, lighting it with a match, and blowing out the match, as regards both the succession of the individual acts and the skill in the movements.

BUCCOFACIAL APRAXIA. *Wrinkling her brows*: She moves her eyes uncertainly, lifts up her head. Urged, she wrinkles her brows a little; continuously urged she does so more distinctly; but now at the same time she moves her lower jaw. *Closing her eyes*: She does so, but simultaneously nods her head. *Turning up her nose*: She closes her eyes, moves her cheeks a little. When shown how to do it, she inclines her head and casts down her eyes, but does not perform any movement of the nose. *Sneezing*: Draws air in through the nose and pushes it out through the mouth. When shown how to do it, she moves her head, then she utters some sounds that are similar to coughing and hawking. *Pursing up her lips*: She opens her mouth a little. When shown how to do it, she wrinkles her brows and opens her mouth. When emphatically shown how to do it, she nods her head and opens her mouth. *Whistling*: Does it correctly. For this act she purses her lips very well, though she was not able to do so just before. *Puffing her cheeks*: She moves her lips. When shown how to do it, she opens her mouth, moves her brows and eyes. *Blowing*: She whistles. When she is told to do as if she were blowing out a candle, she whistles again. When a burning match is held in front of her she immediately blows it out correctly. *Showing her teeth*: She moves the lower jaw forward a little, then slightly purses her lips. *Protruding her tongue*: She moves her lips and uncertainly her cheeks. When urged she by and by protrudes her tongue. *Placing her tongue to the right*: Instead she moves her tongue back again. *Clearing her throat*: Wrinkles her brows, opens her eyes wide, then hawks in a low voice but correctly. *Coughing*: She instead clears her throat. When urged to do it properly, she moves her head and even her shoulders, and hawks again. When shown how to do it, she approximately succeeds.

Looking to the right or to the left was impossible on command. But when her head was held fast and the direction was shown with the finger, then she succeeded in looking to the sides. Whistling, which she had carried out correctly one day, could not be performed on another day.

SPEECH. *Understanding*: In conversation the patient understood every word immediately. Named objects were shown by her at once if they were within her visual field; otherwise she would look around her, until she saw them. She found the pocket-lamp though hidden behind records, remarking: 'It surely was here just now.' With the exception of the fingers, the parts of her body were generally shown correctly after being named; but yet slight difficulties seemed to exist. She did not point at once to her elbow but by way of her breast. To the hollow of her knee she pointed by way of the calf of her leg. Her right ankle was not shown by her at all; instead she pointed to the knee, then to her shin-bone.

Repetitive speech. Bäcker (baker): 'Bä ... Bäck ... Bä ... Bäcker, eben (just).' *Tischtuch* (table-cloth): 'Gi ... Tische ... Tisch ... Tischto ... Tischtoch ... Tisch.' Once more *Tischtuch:* 'Tischto ...' *Tuch* (cloth): Correctly repeated. *Tisch* (table): Correctly repeated. *Wand* (wall): Correctly repeated. *Schrank* (cup-board): 'Schra ... kann ich nicht (I cannot) ... Sch ... Tisch ...' Once more *Schrank*: 'Sch ... aa ... Sch ... nein, kann nicht (no, cannot).' *Kleid* (dress): 'Fei ... Ha ... Schel ...' Once more *Kleid*: 'Scha ... ich kann es nicht (I cannot).' She weeps. *Feder* (feather): 'Aa ... aa ... Schö ... Schö ...' Once more *Feder*: 'Schö ... mm ... kann ich nicht (cannot).' *Brille* (spectacles): 'Sch ... Sch ... nein (no).' On another day: *Bleistift* (pencil): 'Stei ... nein (no).' *Tinte* (ink): 'Tin ... Tin ... Tin-te.' *Feder* (feather): 'Fewer ... Fe-ber ... Fe ... Fe-de-der ... Fe ... Fel.' On some days she was more successful. Once she could immediately repeat: *Tischplatte* (table-top), another time: *Ofenrohr* (stove pipe). Words that she did not know she could never repeat. *Andra*: 'Deck ... Deck ...'. *Poly*: 'Pe ... pe ... pe ...'.

In spontaneous speech the patient articulated the single sounds correctly. However, sometimes she could not correctly repeat single sounds on command. In saying the alphabet she said 'P', 'S' and 'T' instead of 'G'. Only when she had repeated 'Gans' (goose) correctly did she succeed in saying 'G'. Similar difficulties arose in connection with 'H' and 'S', though she had before said 'S' instead of 'G'.

Reading: *Klinik* (clinic): 'Ke ... Ke ... Keve ... Kli ... Klinik.' *Babette*: 'End ... End ... Ende ...' *Krankengeschichte* (record): 'Krank ... Kranken ... Kranken ...'

Naming: *Rose* (rose): 'Ro ... Rose.' *Taschenlampe* (pocket-lamp): 'La ... Lam ... Lampe.' *Gummi* (rubber): 'Hug ... Hug ... Gu ... Lung ... sehen Sie da (you can see) ... La ... Lang ... (fingers the rubber permanently) La ... was ist denn – mit mir (what is the matter – with me).' *Bleistift* (pencil): 'Ble ... Bler ... Ble ... Blei.' *Notizbuch* (notebook): 'Ble ... für (for) Ble ... Ble ... Blei ... für zum (for) Blei.' *Papierkorb* (wastepaper basket): 'Zum (for) ... Kast ... zur (for) ... sch ...' She weeps. *Federhalter* (penholder): 'Tif ... Tif ...'. Once more *Federhalter*: 'Ho ... Tri ....' Once more *Federhalter*: 'Sto ... St ... Herr Doktor, ich kann doch nichts dafür, das kommt doch wieder? (Doctor, it is not my fault, will it be cured?)' She weeps. – 'Es hat ha ... hat sich schon sehr se ... sehr gut, gut g ... g ...' (it is much better already). *Tintenfass* (inkstand): 'A ... Ding ... aa ... zum (for) ... für zu (for) ... Gestern abend hat erst mein Mann ... noch gesagt, Frau musst dich ... mehr lernen (Only yesterday evening my husband ... said, you must ... learn more).' Again and again she, wanting help, touches the inkstand. – On another day: *Füller* (fountain-pen): 'Fillge ... Gle ... Pfe ... Filt ... Tilt.' *Buch* (book): 'Eh ... eh ... na ... na ... Bu ... Buch.' *Klammer* (clip): 'Tran ... Tran ... Klammer.' *Brille* (spectacles): 'Br ... Br ... Bringe ... Bringe ... ach als wieder (ah, again).'

Spontaneous speech: The patient speaks almost nothing of her own accord. To questions she gives her personal data, speaks of her state of health and her second marriage, and in this she is able to speak several sentences without difficulties. But attempting to enter into general conversation, the breaks set in. – (How long have you been married?) 'I cannot say ... now this happened, and I am living still ... I have not ... not at all ... What is the matter with me? ... I have a boy.' (What school does he attend?) 'He goes to ... na ... he has done something ... together with other children ... He has ... yes ... I cannot ...' (What does he learn?) 'Bett ... Metzger (butcher) ...

Bätz ... Bäck ...' (Bäcker?) 'Yes.' (Does he learn easily?) 'Yes he has always ge ... ge ...' (Been). 'Yes, quite well.'

Articulation: If the correct word or the right syllable was pronounced, the articulation was fully correct. However, the wrong sounds, which the patient wanted to withdraw immediately, often were slurred.

In this patient (after arteriosclerotic encephalomalacia), we found many parietal lobe symptoms: right–left confusion, finger agnosia, constructional apraxia, dysgraphia, dyslexia, acalculia, and temporal disorientation. The narrowing of the visual field showed that deeper subcortical areas were destroyed. Another parietal symptom, clearly evident, was the severe ideokinetic apraxia of the hands and of the face. This form of apraxia is demonstrated by the movements permanently slipping (derailing), and is confirmed by the movements being correctly performed in real situations when handling actual objects.

Besides, there was a very severe motor aphasia. Sensory aphasic disorders were absent. The slight difficulties of the patient in showing the parts of her body were related to finger agnosia and had no aphasic basis. Sensory aphasia was apparently never present because from the beginning only a disorder of pronunciation was mentioned. In our examination we found enormous difficulties in forming words. Repetition and naming were grossly impaired. Frequently in short words, regularly in longer words, the patient, after beginning to speak, stopped and began anew. Again and again she began and stopped. Sometimes the first phoneme was the only correct sound, sometimes it was different from what the patient wished to pronounce. The incorrect sounds then were repeated or other incorrect sounds appeared. From time to time the patient finally succeeded in uttering the complete word. Usually the incorrect syllables resembled the correct ones, but sometimes, especially after a fruitless endeavour, quite different syllables appeared. In this case we were reminded of the paraphasias of sensory aphasia, but the patient really knew which word she wanted to say and was only unsuccessful in pronouncing it. We were sometimes reminded also of amnestic aphasia, especially when the patient tried to replace a word which she could not pronounce by another word with similar meaning. But the difference from an amnestic disorder could easily be recognized, since the patient was also unable to pronounce the circumlocutory word she

22

had chosen herself. Moreover, the possibility of an amnestic disorder is disproved by the fact that in repetition, when the complete word was said to her, the patient had even more difficulties than when naming. There is no doubt that the disorder was a pure motor aphasia.

However, if the patient was successful, the speech was fluent, not slow, and not laboured. The breaks were not due to difficulties in articulation, but only arose when the patient observed that she had pronounced a wrong sound, which was to be corrected, or if she anticipated that an incorrect word would appear. Her incidental remarks confirmed the origin of the breaks: after a wrong syllable had appeared, she would indicate that she was sorry; moreover, she was disappointed when trying in vain to pronounce the correct syllable. So the regulation of the speech movements was disturbed, not the articulation.

In acting the patient showed the same inability as in speaking. If she wanted to pronounce a word, she began, stopped, began again, deviated into a wrong sound, began again and usually derailed again. Just in the same way on command she began to move her hand, deviated into a wrong movement, stopped, tried to move correctly, and usually did not succeed. The same behaviour was also observed in relation to movements of the face, the lips, and the tongue, so that it may be said that in oral apraxia and in aphasia the same muscles (including the velar and laryngeal muscles) worked incorrectly in the same manner.

There is another parallel. As is well known, ideokinetic apraxia does not become apparent in actions performed in situations to which the patient has become accustomed. It appears only when actions are to be performed without a direct concrete referent. Liepmann (1900) explained this plausibly by a short cut of everyday movements in natural situations. It is desirable to distinguish an apraxia with actual objects from an apraxia without such objects, as indicated by some authors (see Zangwill, 1960; De Renzi, Pieczuro and Vignolo, 1968; Heilman, 1973). Ideational apraxia should not be mixed in for it is a disturbance not of the single act but of the sequence and accretion of several acts. This is a major difference. A patient suffering from ideational apraxia who fails in lighting a candle perhaps holds the match to the candle, without first striking it, or tries to strike it on the candle or on the wrong side of the matchbox. However, the act of striking the match in itself is executed correctly, and the patient is also able to perform this movement correctly upon command, without the actual candle. In this way do classical as well as modern authors (Ajuriaguerra and Hécaen, 1960; Ajuriaguerra and Tissot, 1969) describe ideational apraxia. Perhaps ideational apraxia is not a genuine apraxia but the result of a defect of memory.

Surely we can follow Liepmann's explanation. Therefore, if we, in concert with Kleist, regard ideokinetic apraxia as a kinesthetic disorder, we can suppose that the movements which are habitualized from everyday situations no longer require kinesthetic checking, but are sufficiently organized in the innervatory sphere to be performed automatically. On the other hand, when by unusual arrangements the automatic action is deranged, the disturbance arises, for example when the patient is asked to turn a coffee grinder, or to threaten without a naughty child being present, or to salute without being a soldier. Our patient performed correct movements if the movements were based upon an actual situation and were not merely abstract. The same holds true regarding her facial apraxia. She was unable to blow without something to blow, but blew out a candle quite correctly. She could not purse her lips on command but pursed them correctly in whistling. Another day she could not whistle, obviously because the automatism had failed.

Similarly, in the aphasia of our patient spontaneous speech is least affected. From the normal desire to have a talk, from the momentary context of thoughts in speaking, automaticity works best. Therefore spontaneously very much can be spoken without breaks; kinesthetic regulation to a certain degree is not necessary here; innervatory organization is sufficient.

It is the same phenomenon that explains why our patient, who could articulate all sounds, sometimes was unable to speak on command the most simple sounds, for instance *G* or *S*. Even here the automatism was not efficient enough to articulate on command. And again, the phenomenon is presented by our patient's inability to cough and clear her throat upon command, although she coughed and cleared her throat spontaneously very often. The statement that some sounds, which the patient wanted to withdraw immediately, were slurred is explained by her attempts to suppress or to correct the wrong sound. In short: Moving in apraxia as well as speaking in aphasia were disturbed predominantly upon command, but much less in spontaneous production.

24

Repetition was not easier for the patient than naming, nor was imitation easier than acting without being shown how to do it. It was of no use to demonstrate to the patient how to perform an action; her failure was quite the same as before.

The speech of our patient thus exhibits the same disturbance as her motor acts and, what is more, it exhibits only this disturbance. The speech is ideokinetically apractic, cannot follow the directions that are sensorily correctly given. There is no further disorder.

Case No. 2. Wilhelm Elb., born in 1897, mason. In the summer of 1948 he had an accident. He fell about two metres down from a scaffold and struck his head upon a roller. He was not unconscious, but consulted a physician and was certified as ill because of bruises. After several weeks he worked again. In December, 1949 he became ill again. He suddenly felt sick, fell down and was unconscious for some time. Upon regaining consciousness he had no strength and no feeling in the right arm and could no longer speak. In February, 1950 he was admitted to the hospital. He complained of difficulties in speaking and of clumsiness of the right hand. There was a little cardiac murmur and a tachycardia. Electrocardiogram showed an infirmity of the myocardium and a sinus arhythmia. Speech was a little slurred, the right hand showed a trembling. Oppenheim's and Gordon's sign could be elicited on the right side. A bulbar paralysis was suspected. In October, 1950 the consulted neurologist found apraxia of the face, tongue, and arms, in addition to an antagonistic tremor of the arms.

In August and October, 1951 the patient was in the Frankfurt/ Main clinic, where I examined him. He told me that even before the attack in December, 1949 he had headaches and difficulties in speaking. After the fainting spell his condition had become worse, but then had stabilized.

There was a slight lividity of the lips, a tachycardia of 104 pulsations, and a blood-pressure of 145/95. The right corner of the mouth was a little deeper than the left. An attempt to show the teeth blocked initially. Mimicking was stiff. The arms, especially the right arm, showed a tremor in relaxation, and increasingly so when the arms were stretched forward. There was a rigidity in the right arm. The strength of the right hand was a little reduced; periosteal reflexes were a little increased. In the legs there was no disturbance regarding strength, tone and tendon reflexes. Gordon's sign could be elicited on the right side. Sensibility was intact in all parts of the body. The electroencephalogram was normal.

Elb. was somewhat depressed in reaction to his severe illness. Orientation as to time and to place was intact. There was no visual agnosia, no finger agnosia, no acalculia. In reading of some words the same difficulties arose as in repetition. Other disorders of reading could not be found. He fully understood what he read. Writing was not possible because of the tremor.

APRAXIA OF THE HANDS. *Threatening, left hand*: He makes a full fist, moves his hand uncertainly during which he opens his fist again, moves his fingers. *Right hand*: He makes a fist. *Threatening with the left forefinger*: He first stretches his forefinger forward, then all fingers, then moves his hand to and fro. When shown how to do it, he partly bends his fingers, then stretches them again and continues moving his flat hand to and fro. *Beckoning, left hand*: The movements are more striking than beckoning, the fingers are partly stretched, partly bent. *Right hand*: He alternately opens and closes his hand. When shown how to do it, he makes a gesture that resembles the correct response. *Knocking, left hand*: He knocks with the finger-tips on the wall, then a little better with the back of the fingers. *Asked to do so even better*: He now rubs the back of the fingers at the wall. *Saluting*: He, on the right as well as on the left, lays the whole flat hand at the temple. *Turning a coffee grinder, left hand*: He moves the hand first uncertainly to and fro, then gradually performs circular movements, but holds the fingers simply stretched. *Right hand*: He closes the hand a little, but then, instead of circular movements, he performs movements of catching. *Putting on a hat*: He first moves his closed fist to his head, then his flat hand without performing the requested specific movements. Invited to put on the cap that lies beside him, he immediately does so with wholly correct and natural movements.

BUCCOFACIAL APRAXIA. *Closing his eyes*: Correct. *Open again*: Correct. *Turning his eyes to the right*: He turns his head. When shown how to do it, he repeatedly moves his head a little to the right and returns; the eyes are not moved. *Moving his eyes down*: He stoops his head. When his head is held fast, then his eyes move downward transiently and incompletely. *Following a moving finger with his eyes*: He does this correctly, only sometimes a little slowly. *Wrinkling his brows*: His eyes move uncertainly. When shown how to do it, he moves his lips but not his brows. *Closing his eyes tightly*: He closes his eyes but, in spite of repeated encouraging and showing how to do it, he does not close them tightly. *Turning up his nose*: He performs movements with his lips, protrudes his tongue, contracts the wings of his nose. When shown how to do it, he snaps with his mouth and then keeps the mouth open. *Opening his mouth*: He opens and shuts his mouth, and between these movements he protrudes his tongue. When shown how to do it, he performs movements resembling licking and smacking. *Puffing his cheeks*: He performs uncertain movements with his tongue and his mouth, in addition to movements of his arms. *Blowing*: He performs uncertain movements of the mouth. When shown how to do it, he first uncertainly moves cheeks and lips, then produces a movement resembling a short blowing. *Protruding his tongue*: The tongue several times licks over the lips, but each time returns at once into the cavity of the mouth. When shown how to do it, movements of the head appear, in addition to the licking.

SPEECH. Understanding was completely intact. Even when the topics of conversation were rapidly changed, the patient understood immediately. Special examinations confirmed his intact understanding.

Repetition: Short words are repeated correctly. *Tischtuch* (Table-cloth): 'Tisch-tuch.' *Matrazenpolster* (mattress-bolster): 'Bat ... baza-polser ... Mat-ratz-polster ....' *Bettstelle* (bedstead): 'Bettich ... Betsche ... Betelle ....' *Bettfedern* (bed-feather): 'Bett-federn.' *Türklinke* (door-handle): 'Kir ... Kir-klinke ... Türklinke.' *Berufs-genossenschaft* (professional association): 'Berufs-nossenschaft ... Berufs-nossen-fasch ... Berufs-nissen-haff ... Berufs-do-nos–haft ... Berufs-nossen-haff.' *Magistratsrat* (municipal officer): 'Mag-rat ... Madi-vatis-rat ... Magi-rat ... Rat.' *Schiffahrtsgesellschaft* (shipping company): 'Schiff-rat-g-schaft ... Fisch-fahrt-gessel-schaft ... Fisch-art-selart ... Fisch-fahrt-fahrt ... Gessel-schaft.' *Donauschiff* (Danube-ship): 'Donau-sched ... dona-schiff ... Donausch-schiff ... Donauschiff.' *Reichstagsabgeordneter* (Parliament delegate): 'Reichstag-ab-ordnet ... Reichstagsab-e-ordet ... Reichstags-ab-de-ordnet.' *Abgeordneter* (delegate): 'Abgeordnet ... Abgeord-et ... Abge-ordne-ter.'

The following Greek words could not be understood by the patient. These words, as well as the former words, were said before the patient time and again, while he tried to repeat them. – *Anthropos*: 'Antosch-pos ... antra-os.' *Enepe*: 'Eweke ... enke ... ennep-pe ... enelpe ... ene-ke.' *Pola*: 'Ola ... pola.' *Angelo*: 'Ankelor.' *Paitomai*: 'Paitonait ... paite-nait'. *Domai*: 'Damai ... dama ... demoi ... do-mai.'

Naming: Short names are given correctly. *Stehlampe* (standard lamp): 'Elektrisch ... Steh-lap ... Stehlampe.' *Armbanduhr* (wrist-watch): 'Uhr'. When requested to be more precise: 'Arm-buhr ... Arm ... bnd-buhr ... Amba-dir.' *Selbstbinder* (open-end tie): 'Selbstr-bindr ... Selbster-bindr.' *Schreibtisch* (writing-table): 'Tisch ... Reit-tisch ....'

Spontaneous speech: The patient did not speak much, often stopped, but articulated some other words rapidly. Occasionally in spontaneous speech he was obliged to correct himself, because he had erred in forming a word. He tried to express himself in short sentences, but did not avoid the grammatical connections and used them correctly.

Articulation: Some words were slurred so that they could not be well understood. This seemingly happened when the patient tried quickly to get past an anticipated error in forming a word which was about to appear. Generally he spoke a little slowly. Single phonemes were all normally articulated. Perhaps the articulation was a little affected by the brain stem lesion, which was proved by the tremor, the rigidity, and the slight mimic disorder. As a slight tremor was also to be found in the left hand, the right hemisphere was probably involved too. The etiology of the illness could not be exactly clarified; one or two embolisms resulting from a cardiac disorder may be assumed.

The brain stem lesion did not influence the symptomatology very much. Only writing could not be examined because of the tremor. Ideokinetic apraxia could be appreciated also in the right hand, despite the trembling. Finer movements were sufficiently well performed with the left hand.

Compared with the first patient, Elb. appears less affected, but his syndrome is purer because further parietal lobe symptoms are missing. Again there is a combination of very characteristic apraxic and aphasic disturbances. The gross deviations into wrong movements, arising in apraxia of the arms as well as of the face, prove the ideokinetic form. In speaking we find the slips into wrong sounds and syllables, which are noticed at once and corrected, unless a new slip occurs. In repetition and naming the disturbance is severe, in spontaneous speech slighter. Furthermore the patient spoke slowly and haltingly, separating the single sounds and syllables. The breaks only partly corresponded to the natural separations within the words. Often the speech broke off in the middle of a syllable.

Case No. 3. Walter Jas., born in 1916, butcher. He was wounded on the upper edge of the left temple in 1941. He was paralyzed on the right side and could not speak for three months. Shortly afterwards epileptic fits began and have recurred from time to time ever since. In 1944 a clinical record read: 'The motor aphasia has very much changed for the better. The vocabulary and the formation of sentences are still restricted.' The radiographic findings were: 'On the left side in the coronal suture a small defect of the bone is to be seen, around which some small bone splinters are visible. A larger shell-splinter, approximately the shape of an infantry projectile, lies deep in the skull, near the median line, about four centimetres above the sella turcica.' The encephalographic findings were: 'Slight enlargement of all ventricles without special topical displacement or dilatation. The metal splinter is very near the wall of the third ventricle.'

In January and February 1947, and in June and July 1952, the patient was treated in the infirmary for brain diseases (Hirnverletztenheim) in Bad Homburg. In 1947 mention is made of some paraphasias. In 1952 I examined and treated the patient in the infirmary. The examination revealed that the hemiplegia of the right hand was almost complete, while the right facial nerve was paretic, there was a spastic paretic gait on the right side and hypesthesia in all qualities on the right side. Understanding of speech, calculating, constructing were intact. The patient could read very well and write with the left hand sufficiently well. Vigor, productivity and concentration were decreased, but memory and intelligence were intact. There were epileptic fits every few weeks.

PRAXIA OF THE LEFT HAND (the right arm is paralytic). *Beckoning to approach*: He lifts his arm and moves his fingers uncertainly. *Threatening*: He stretches his forefinger forward and then moves his hand clumsily. *Knocking*: He brings his forefinger to the correct position, but then threatens. On a second trial, he swings his hand to and fro, but the movements are now a little closer to knocking. *Saluting* is correctly carried out. *Taking off his hat*: He holds the hand correctly beside the head, but does not proceed in taking off the hat; then simply lets his hand down. When shown how to do it, he simply repeats his former movements. *Turning a coffee grinder*: He does so correctly, except that he describes the circle much too widely. When shown how to do it, the circle becomes a little smaller but still remains much too wide. *Thumbing his nose*: He does so correctly, except that he holds his hand too far from his nose. *Polishing shoes*: He first rotates his hand strangely, then he moves it to and fro, but without the movement of polishing being recognizable. *Eating soup*: He first moves the hand uncertainly to and fro, then towards the face, but the specific movement of using a spoon is not recognizable. *Playing the violin*: He makes a fist and moves it to and fro.

It should be noted that the patient always handles actual objects correctly. Also finer movements in real situations such as buttoning his clothes or playing the piano are correctly carried out.

BUCCOFACIAL APRAXIA. *Wrinkling his brows*: He raises his brows a little, then moves them uncertainly. When shown how to do it, he raises his head but not his brows. *Closing his eyes*: He closes his eyes, but opens them again immediately. *Turning his eyes to the right*: He moves his head more than his eyes to the right. After several attempts he succeeds even less; finally he only moves his head, with no eye movement at all. He fails equally in his attempts to turn his eyes to the left, upwards, or downwards. *Showing his teeth*: He does it correctly but not forcibly. *Whistling*: He blows. *Puffing his left cheek*: He puffs both cheeks. When shown how to do it, he again puffs both cheeks and turns his mouth a little to the left. *Puffing his right cheek*: He again puffs both cheeks. *Protruding his tongue*: Correct. *Moving his tongue upwards*: In trying to do so he, instead, moves his tongue backwards. *Clearing his throat*: He does not succeed. When shown how to do it, he produces a croaking sound. When shown a second time, he produces a sound a little closer to the target. *Coughing*: Correct. *Sneezing*: He blows through his nose without producing the characteristic sound of sneezing.

SPEECH. *Repetition*: *Tintenfass* (inkstand): Correct. *Fensterrahmen* (window frame): 'Fensteram'. When requested to articulate better: 'Fenster-Fenster-ram'. *Matratzenschoner* (spring cover): 'Ma-trat-zen-schoner'. *Türklinke* (door-handle): 'Tür-klinke'. *Handwerks-bursche* (travelling craftsman): Many breaks between the single sounds. *Laubbaum* (tree with foliage): Breaks between the syllables.

Handwerksmeister (master craftsman) 'Hand-werks-meister'. *Flannel-lapen* (flannel duster): 'S ... S ... kann ich nicht (cannot) ... sa ... sa ... sam.' *Schellfisch* (haddock): He begins several times but does not succeed. After the word has been pronounced by the examiner several times and after he himself has made several attempts, he finally succeeds in speaking the word slowly and with several breaks. *Gesellschaft* (society): 'Ge-sell ... Geschell ... Ge-sell-schaft.'

Naming: He pronounces quite slowly but names correctly. Sometimes he begins to name only after a pause. Sometimes he replaces a word: *Tintenfass* (inkstand): 'Where the ink is put in, Tintenfass.' Sometimes he deforms a word: *Indianer* (Indian): 'Ital ... Italianer ... In ... Ind-dianer.'

This patient, in a less distinct form, showed the symptoms that were found in the other two cases. The ideokinetic apraxia of the hands and of the face was still evident. The language was less disturbed, but in difficult words the disorder was still recognizable, in repetition more than in naming. However, it must be noted that in repetition most of the desired words were much longer and more difficult than the words used in naming. In spontaneous speech paraphasias did not occur at all. But this surely is due to the fact that the patient avoided words that he could not easily pronounce and instead substituted others. This disorder resembled an amnestic aphasic disturbance, but, just as in our first case, only the motor finding of the word was in fact difficult. In all forms of speech, also in spontaneous speech, we found hesitant production, continuously slowed down by short interruptions, which could also be observed in Patient No. 2. In the first patient (Fel.) this manner of speaking was not significant, but probably only because she again and again slipped and was obliged to stop. While improving, the patients are able to avoid paraphasias by carefully preparing every syllable. They in consequence cannot speak fluently. Halting speech, slowed by breaks, therefore arouses the suspicion of ideokinetic aphasia, or of residual influences of this form of aphasia. The lesser degree of disturbance in patient Jas. is understandable since the injury had occurred twelve years before my examination took place. So there was much time for compensation. The aphasia had improved more than the apraxia. This is not astonishing, since language was more necessary and in consequence had received more effort. The apraxic disorder does not appear in real situations and is often only discovered in neuro-psychological examinations. Thanks to the short cut, mentioned earlier, everyday movements remain possible.

The described cases clinically demonstrate that an ideokinetic form of aphasia exists. It is unlikely that the characteristic disturbance should arise by combination of two different disorders; for the aphasia shows quite the same features as the apraxia. Just as in apraxia the correct movements are not found by the patients and breaks and slips into incorrect movements occur, so in aphasia the correct speech movements are not found and breaks and slips into wrong sounds and syllables follow. If it is true that in ideokinetic apraxia the kinesthetic patterns of the movements have been lost, then in the described aphasia the kinesthetic patterns of the speech movements no longer exist. The differences decrease even more when we consider within apraxia those movements which are combined with sounds, such as coughing, clearing the throat, or sneezing. If the movement is not found ideokinetically, incorrect sounds arise just as in aphasia.

However, the conformity of apraxia with aphasia does not mean that the lesions producing them must be located precisely in the same area of the brain. On the one hand, apraxia of the limbs arises from a different region than apraxia of the face; the regions are adjacent, however. On the other hand, for the extremely important sphere of speaking a separate cortical area would be expected to be necessary, though some of the same muscles are used. The understanding of melodies is not disturbed by damage to the region involved in the understanding of speech. It is even possible that buccofacial apraxia and apraxia of speech sometimes depend on different hemispheres, in the same way that amusia is sometimes produced by lesions of the minor hemisphere, whereas, at the same time, speech is intact. I once saw a singer who seemingly suffered from ideokinetic amusia. He knew, he said, distinctly which tone he was to sing, but he could not produce it. He had no aphasia, but a slight facial apraxia. Because the disturbance improved rather quickly, I could not examine this very interesting feature more thoroughly.

Some authors are of the opinion that the more primitive functions are generally dependent upon lesions in the right, the more complicated functions upon lesions in the left hemisphere. Henschen (1920–1922), Jackson (1932), Nielsen (1946) and many others relate emotional speech to the minor hemisphere. Accordingly, facial

32

apraxia, the more primitive function, may in some cases arise from lesions in the minor hemisphere. However, this may be even more true regarding innervatory apraxia. The cases of Domnick (1943), mentioned earlier, had lesions predominantly in the right hemisphere. As regards facial apraxia as well as ideokinetic aphasia, the cases described above were associated with lesions in the left hemisphere. In some other cases I saw ideokinetic aphasia without apraxia or the latter without aphasia. So, at any rate, a lesion of exactly the same region may not produce both disturbances; but it is undecided whether in these cases the minor hemisphere was responsible for apraxia or whether the lesion was so small that of the two adjoining areas only one was destroyed.

If one considers ideokinetic aphasia a separate form of aphasia, the question arises as to how it is related to the aphasias described so far. In my opinion, most cases of so called conduction aphasia are not produced by disconnection, but by cortical lesions of the parietal lobe, though the breaks and the slips of speech are not accurately described in this type of aphasia. The patient of Goldstein (1914) as well as the cases of Kleist (1934) seem to demonstrate the parietal impairment. All cases of so called conduction aphasia should be examined for ideokinetic apraxia. In many cases apraxia is mentioned but the authors do not regard it as important.

However, there is another kind of conduction aphasia, which is found in the course of recovery from sensory aphasia, first described by Liepmann and Pappenheim (1914). It is extremely important to separate this special form from ideokinetic aphasia. The patients in this stage are no longer sensory aphasics, i.e. their understanding is intact again, but they still show paraphasias. Contrary to the ideokinetic aphasic patients, they speak freely and of their own accord. They need not be encouraged. While speaking fluently they usually notice their errors later than do ideokinetic aphasics, i.e. only when the words are completely pronounced. They rarely interrupt the pronunciation of an incorrect sound, in order to correct it. This is a characteristic difference from ideokinetic aphasics, who at the outset of speech notice their mistakes and try to correct them. Because of this starting and stopping, the speech of these patients is very wearisome. In order to demonstrate the differences I quote the utterances of a patient suffering from conduction aphasia after sensory aphasia.

.   .   .

Case No. 4. Babette Grei. *Naming*: *Brille* (spectacles): 'Der Brill.'
Armbanduhr (wrist-watch): 'Armbuhr.' *Ring* (ring): 'Der Ringe.'
Notizbuch (notebook): 'Buch.' When requested to be more precise:
'Butes, alles muss es wiss' ('butes'=neologism, 'es' instead of 'er',
'wiss' instead of 'wissen'). *Schreibtisch* (writing desk): 'Das ist
Tisch.' When requested to be more precise: 'Zum Grei der Grein-
tisch.' *Schreibmaschine* (type-writer): 'Das ist die Freund ... Das
kann ich jetzt nicht aussprechen (I now cannot pronounce that).'
Tintenfass (inkstand): 'Die Tinte.' When requested to be more
precise: 'Tintenbuch.' *Tintenbuch?*: 'Ach, jetzt dumm ... Tintenfoch.'
Fläschchen (small bottle): 'Ansensis.' *What does that mean?* 'Mates
(=neologism).'

    Repetition: *Seifenschälchen* (soap-dish): 'Seiche ... How often I
have said it so well by myself and now I cannot pronounce.' *Schreibmaschine* (type-writer): 'Seder ... zum Aus ... s-s-sch-schwe ...' *Taschenlampe* (pocket-lamp): 'Tasselbanke.' Once more *Taschenlampe*:
'Sie Tank ... die Tansche ... yes if someone goes away.' *Bettuch*
(sheet): 'Gettuch, Bettuch.' *Ofenrohr* (stove pipe): 'Osenohr-Ohr-
Ohr.' Once more *Ofenrohr*: 'Oses-Ohr-Os-Ohr.' *Tintenfass* (inkstand): 'Tentes.'

If one contrasts this speech with the speech of our ideokinetic patients
the difference becomes obvious. In ideokinetic aphasia we find many
abortive starts, but very rarely full paraphasias. On the contrary
paraphasias are predominant in conduction aphasia. As Patient No. 4
is no longer a sensory aphasic, she notices her errors, as her numerous
incidental remarks show, but usually she cannot stop the words in
due time. Stopping a word at the outset is an exception. We further
recognize readiness of speech, which is typical of this disturbance
whereas ideokinetic aphasics are always sparing in their use of words.

    The disturbance during recovery from sensory aphasia is probably
a genuine conduction disorder. Kleist (1934) explains it by supposing
that the minor hemisphere has learned to understand whereas the
connection with the motor speech area still passes to the dominant
hemisphere and is disturbed there. To the difference in the clinical
picture a difference in the development of the disturbance is added.
Conduction aphasia always follows a sensory aphasia, whereas the
patients with ideokinetic aphasia initially are not able to speak at all.

    Ideokinetic apraxia is a motor disturbance, according to the usual

34

classification. Yet the disorder is produced within a sensory sphere, i.e. within the kinesthetic one, no matter whether we follow the interpretation of Kleist or of Luria. The same holds true in respect to ideokinetic aphasia. In the kinesthetic sphere a pattern (Kleist, 1934) or an integration (Luria, 1966) is disturbed which normally would make possible the correct transmission of sounds, syllables, and words to the motor sphere. In accordance with the classical view one should say that the kinesthetic images of speaking are lost. But, whatever theoretical conception one adopts, the parallel between ideokinetic apraxia and ideokinetic aphasia demonstrates that both disorders are produced by the same damage to a certain region of the brain or to adjacent areas. Ideokinetic apraxia results from lesions of the supramarginal gyrus of the parietal lobe. This has been stated by Liepmann, Kleist and many others. Consequently ideokinetic aphasia is a *parietal aphasia*. I have upheld this view for more than twenty years (Leonhard, 1954), although anatomical confirmation could only be given by Schulze in 1965.

The connection with ideokinetic apraxia as well as the localization in the parietal lobe must be considered when we seek the relationship with classical motor aphasia, i.e. Broca's aphasia. This form of aphasia seems to comprise a disorder corresponding to innervatory apraxia, and to include dysarthria. But in Broca's aphasia, except for stereotyped words, nothing can be said at all. Such speech reduction cannot be produced by dysarthria alone. In ideokinetic aphasia speech is completely impossible in the beginning, but is recovered later on. It is easy to understand that the faculty of speech cannot be restored if there are disturbances in the kinesthetic as well as in the motor sphere. In fact, I am of the opinion that Broca's aphasia is composed of two types of motor impairment-dysarthria on the one hand, and ideokinetic aphasia on the other.

Anatomical findings support this view. Even in Broca's own cases the lesions extended to the parietal lobe. This holds true for later observations as well. Conrad (1948) reports that in Broca's aphasia one has always found large lesions. Obviously two areas are involved, the area affected in dysarthria, i.e. the third frontal convolution, as well as the area affected in ideokinetic aphasia, i.e. the supramarginal convolution. So, not only the clinical but also the anatomical findings seem to indicate that Broca's aphasia is produced by a combination of dysarthria and ideokinetic aphasia.

35

Though most authors at present are of the opinion that Broca's aphasia should not, clinically and anatomically, be considered an entity, they probably will disagree with the conception expressed above. Bay, for one, considers a disorder of conceptual thinking to be the basis of aphasia, when language impairment is more than simple dysarthria. On the other hand, Lhermitte and Gautier (1969) hold Broca's aphasia to be a combination of Wernicke's aphasia and of anarthria. Probably the latter opinion is due to the fact that paraphasias are generally regarded as sensory. Regarding localization, Lhermitte and Gautier refer to the third frontal convolution, the posterior part of the first temporal convolution and the isthmus linking the parietal and occipital lobes with the basal ganglia and insular region. As may be seen, they include even Wernicke's region but neglect the parietal lobe, as do so many other authors. To be sure, they do mention the investigations of Penfield and Roberts (1959) who established the areas necessary for speaking by electrical stimulation of the cerebral cortex during surgical intervention in conscious patients. They reprint a figure from Penfield and Roberts, and two pages earlier a figure originally set forth by Dejerine (1914). We can see very clearly that the latter classical author knew only the centres in the temporal and in the frontal lobe, whereas by electrical stimulation the parietal lobe was added as important for speech. In modern publications about aphasia the parietal lobe is mentioned more often than formerly but not nearly as often as would be desirable. *For the function of speech and for the understanding of the disorders of speech the parietal lobe is as important as the temporal lobe and is even more important than the frontal lobe, damage to which does not produce aphasia in a strict sense but rather dysarthria.*

2. *Ideokinetic aphasia in audiomutism*
Much attention has been paid in recent years to aphasia and apraxia in children (Alajouanine and Lhermitte, 1965; Berges, 1966). Formerly neurologists thought that neuropsychological disturbances in children had to be judged differently from those of adults. This is no longer the usual opinion. Müller (1968) writes that the same disorders can be discussed in childhood, if the function had already developed before the brain injury occurred. Moreover, innate speech disorders, i.e. the different forms of audiomutism, are being increasingly related to aphasia. I leave out of consideration the sensory form, in which the

36

children do not understand speech; I am at the present time concerned only with the motor form. Describing this feature of audio-mutism authors frequently mention a facial apraxia (Tomkiewicz, 1963, 1964; Ajuriaguerra, 1965; Galkowski, 1966; Hasaerts – van Geertruyden, 1966). This characteristic is important.

It is true that many different causes may obtain in cases of children who do not speak though they are not deaf. Schönfelder (1967) made follow-up examinations in 13 children with alleged audiomutism. For some there was a lack of verbal stimulation, others showed a general cerebral disturbance or were imbecilic. Most interesting is the case of a 12 year old boy who showed a faciolingual apraxia. Göllnitz (1958) described apraxia in an audiomute child, and considered the disorder innervatory. In one case (Leonhard, 1954), an ideokinetic form of buccofacial apraxia was found, which could be related to the ideo-kinetic aphasia of the child. Later, together with Berendt and Lindner (1968), I tried to follow audiomute children, but could find only five cases. A patient, now 19 years old, spoke normally; she proved to have suffered from elective mutism. Three patients were severely mentally retarded. In one case we found ideokinetic apraxia and ideokinetic aphasia. I now report the findings in detail.

Case No. 5. Christine F., born 1950, was examined for the first time in 1954 at our mental clinic in Berlin. Intelligence was judged normal. The child understood well, but did not speak at all; she only uttered a few sounds. In 1965 we re-examined the girl, who was then 14 years old.

The mother told us that when the girl was six, speech was so delayed that the teachers refused to allow her to go to a regular school. Persuaded by the mother, school officials yielded and the child began school. By 1965 she had finished the tenth form and was about to become a school nurse.

Patellar reflexes and Achilles tendon reflexes could not be elicited. Otherwise there was no neurological abnormality. In examination of phasia and praxia we found:

Repetition: The patient usually repeated correctly, but haltingly. Sometimes paraphasias occurred, for instance: *Brillenfutteral* (spectacle-case); 'Morillenfutteral'; *Tischdecke* (table-cloth): 'Tischendeck'; *Hausdach* (roof of a house): 'Hausendach'; *Geklopft* (knocked): 'deklopft'; *Konnte* (could); 'Koter'; *Einmal* (once):

37

'Emma'. The patient in any case noticed her mistakes and corrected them on request. Some syllables were pronounced incorrectly. Because this occurred very often, her speech sometimes could not be easily understood. But the patient really was able to pronounce every sound correctly and she did so on request. In such a case she spoke slowly and more haltingly. In spontaneous speech she often had to be told to speak distinctly.

PRAXIA. *Puffing her left cheek*: She moves her mouth to the left and puffs both her cheeks. *Puffing her right cheek*: Same response. Trying in vain to puff her cheek she moves her mouth uncertainly. *Wrinkling her brows*: She lifts her brows a little and at once lowers them again. Urged to keep the brows lifted, she made wrong movements. *Closing one eye*: She always closes both eyes. *Pursing her lips*: After a wrong movement of the lips, the response is correct. *Whistling*: Correct. *Protruding her tongue*: Moves only the tip of her tongue between her teeth. When repeatedly shown how to do it, she once protrudes the tongue strongly, then retracts it. *Turning up her nose*: Does so transiently but together with wrong movements of the forehead. In trying again she adds movements of the corners of her mouth. *Clearing the throat*: Correct. *Coughing*: Does so sufficiently well.

In the arms no apraxia was found, and the fine motor movements of the fingers were not disturbed.

This patient showed signs of brain damage. The ventricles were a little too large and not quite symmetrical. The left cavity was a little bigger than the right. The absence of reflexes in the legs confirmed the structural disturbance. The cause of the enlarged ventricles could not be found.

The speech disorder was characterized by the articulation being intact, when the patient was very careful, while the forming of words was disturbed. This demonstrated the ideokinetic aphasia. As a little child the patient could not speak at all. Later she very laboriously learned to speak but her speech remained defective. Further, there was still a buccofacial apraxia of an ideokinetic nature.

When an adult falls ill with ideokinetic aphasia he does not become mute, but he is no longer able to form words. Speech will be quite impossible if the damage occurs before speech has developed. In the present case there were no syllables which could be connected. Only uncertain phonemes were uttered by the patient at an early age.

38

When she had learned to speak, the feature of ideokinetic aphasia could still be recognized. The patient slipped into wrong sounds and spoke haltingly, as is characteristic in adults with this syndrome.

In more rapid speech, syllables were not well articulated by the patient. In adults with ideokinetic aphasia this occurs when two sounds are about to appear at the same time and merge, before they can be suppressed. In this girl, articulation was much more disturbed. This is surely due to the fact that she had not learned proper articulation earlier. Normally in adults the simple forming of sounds has become automatic and does not require kinesthetic control any longer. The child in learning to speak has to learn at the same time the shaping of the sounds, and therefore Christine F. was not yet skilled in automaticity. With deliberate effort she could articulate each sound, thus demonstrating that there was no disturbance in the innervatory sphere. Contrary to what is observed in cortical dysarthria, articulation was not laboured at all. The buccofacial apraxia confirmed the ideokinetic disturbance by so many slips or wrong movements.

Children suffering from motor audiomutism never learn to speak well, even though understanding is not at all affected and intelligence is good. The functional plasticity of the brain enables a child to acquire fluent speech even when the dominant hemisphere is damaged. In this Roberts (1958) is certainly right. But compensation seems to be impossible if the regions important for speaking are damaged in both hemispheres. This surely was the case in our patient and in other cases of audiomutism in which fluent speech could never be acquired adequately. Other parts of the brain which are not organized for speaking obviously are not able to compensate for such a bilateral deficit. In our patient, the regions responsible for speech in the temporal and frontal lobes probably worked normally, but the region in the parietal lobe was impaired.

3. *Ideokinetic agraphia*

In aphasia classifications, in spite of different opinions, are still primarily determined by classical distinctions. In agraphia, however, we do not find any particular classification to be used widely. This is confirmed by Leischner's careful account (1969). Perhaps the lack of a classificatory system is due to the fact that the relationship between agraphia and apraxia has been neglected. Only Kleist (1934) has paid attention to such a relationship. Liepmann (1900, 1929) in several cases describes a combination of agraphia and apraxia. However, from the severity of the disturbance in these cases we recognize that the patients suffered from an optokinetic form of agraphia, and not from the form related to ideokinetic aphasia. The famous patient of Liepmann (1900) had constructional apraxia, to which the agraphia was related. He had no ideokinetic apraxia. On the other hand, Kleist (1934) mentioned ideokinetic apraxia, but placed more emphasis on a disturbance in pencil handling than on true agraphia. He did mention confusions of letters, however.

Since ideokinetic aphasia is related to conduction aphasia, it is interesting to note the writing disorders which Hécaen and Marcie (1967) found in conduction aphasia. Among other things, they mention literal paragraphias, which are recognized by the patients who then try to correct them. As was pointed out several years ago (Leonhard 1962), this auto-correction is the essential criterion of ideokinetic agraphia. Richter (1962) followed up several cases of ideokinetic aphasia over a long period of time, and in these cases too described a writing disorder. Regarding his first case, Richter made the following remarks: The patient writes his name correctly in block letters. Signature is correct. He always prompts himself as to what he wants to write. *Copying*: Correct. *Dictation*: *Buch* (book): 'Buch'; *Wand* (wall): 'Wande': *Decke* (cover): 'Decke'; *Lampe* (lamp): 'Lampe'; *im Krankenhaus* (in the hospital): 'in im e Kran Klaaden'; *Krankenhaus* (hospital): 'Kran Krangen Kranrenre'; *Zimmer* (room): 'Zimmer'; *Donnerstag* (Thursday): 'Donniwocht Donnerstag'; *22*: '22'; *38*: '38'; *77*: '77'; *198*: '187' (detected and corrected by the patient): '198'.

After some improvement, another examination took place three weeks later: in copying the patient also transcribes errors. Once he leaves out a single letter. Dictated letters and short words can be written, but the patient finds polysyllabic words difficult: *Der Himmel ist stark bewölkt* (the sky is strongly cloudly): 'Der Himmel ist schlast stark bewolgk.' *Die Wiese steht voller Blumen* (the meadow is full of flowers): 'Die Wiese stegt voller Blumen.' His written autobiography consists primarily of incomplete sentences and catchwords with many paragraphias. Short sentences which he forms himself are correctly written with one exception: *Garten* (garden): 'Guarken Guarten.'

About his second case Richter notes that the patient always first tries the correct movement or writes the letter very lightly. Nevertheless he has to correct some letters. He copies slavishly with a shaky hand. *Spontaneous writing*: *Berlin N 4 Bergstr.*: 'Berlin N4, Begstrs.' *Dictation*: Dictated single letters and numbers are correctly written. *Hof* (court): 'Hof'; *König* (king): 'Ko'; *Fenster* (window): 'Fer F'; *Ofenrohr* (stove-pipe): 'Ofen.'

Regarding his third case Richter observes that when copying and writing sentences from dictation the patient makes mistakes. She writes more fluently when she does not pronounce what she wants to write. Confusions are few in writing single letters, and even more rare in writing numerals. *Kleiderbügel* (clothes-horse): 'Kleider Bügel'; *Tabletten* (tablets): 'Tanbletten'; *Türrahmen* (door-frame): 'Türanten'; *Ich bin im Krankenhaus* (I am in hospital): 'in der aus Krankenhaus.' Without prompting herself she writes correctly: 'Ich bin im Krankenhaus.'

Four weeks later: *Copying*: *Der Mond ist aufgegangen, die goldenen Sternlein prangen am Himmel hell und klar* (The moon has risen, the golden stars shine lightly and clearly in the sky): 'Der Mand ist aufgegangen daz Mondel stringen goldnen sternlein prangen am himmel und har (crossed out by the patient) hell und klar.' *Dictation*: *Der Himmel ist stark bewolkt* (The sky is very cloudy): 'Himmel aus dem blaub biw' (crossed out by the patient).

Thus, these patients usually made no mistake when writing isolated letters but confused some letters when writing words. All of them could write their names correctly. But when the first two patients had to write their addresses, errors in the sequence of the letters usually appeared. In each case there were mistakes in the dictations. The third patient often crossed out what she had written, when she had made an error. On the other hand, she confused whole words. The peculiarity is easy to understand when one knows that she was trained in writing. She was a secretary. For this reason not only were single letters habitual to her but also some whole words, which here took the place of letters and consequently were confused.

Similar to the writing of letters was the writing of numbers. Simple digits were written correctly, but the composition of longer numbers often did not turn out well. In two-digit numbers mistakes did not occur, but in three-digit numbers confusions of figures were apparent. Because of this disturbance in the writing of numbers, it was difficult to judge her ability to calculate. For example, when Else B. tried to add 246 and 158, she said correctly that 2 and 1 were 3, but she wrote 1. In mental calculating similar difficulties arose because the patients were also ideokinetic aphasics and failed to speak the numbers correctly. After repeated examinations it could be stated that there was no dyscalculia in patients one and three. In the second case Richter found calculation to be disturbed.

In observing that the patients form the letters correctly but regularly fail in the composition of words, we recognize the parallel to ideokinetic aphasia, in which the articulation of sounds is intact but composition of words not fully possible. When the patients are observed during their writing, we find parallels to the breaks in speech. They stop writing when a wrong letter is about to appear, or has already appeared. The third patient used to cross out incorrect letters, the other two patients usually left the errors and started afresh. However, sometimes they did not stop and seemed not to notice their mistake. So a difference was observed between the way they talked and the way they wrote. In fact, we are much more apt to notice when uttering a wrong syllable than when writing it. In almost every case we notice our slips of the tongue, but we overlook many slips of the pen. So the difference between speaking and writing in the patients' behaviour is certainly not essential. When the patients were asked whether their writing was correct, they read it over and recognized confusions of letters in each case. Moreover, it could sometimes be seen from the patient's countenance that he had noticed a mistake, but failed to correct it because it was troublesome.

Richter discusses the possibility that paragraphias might be the simple result of incorrect speaking, i.e. they might be written paraphasias. But this is easily refuted. A slip in speaking, noticed immediately by the patients, will never be repeated in writing. The term 'written paraphasia' means that a word is first wrongly spoken and later on wrongly written. This frequently occurs in sensory aphasics, who do not recognize their mistakes. Our patients, since they take pains not to pronounce a word incorrectly, will certainly decline to write it. Furthermore, some written words cannot be pronounced at all. Several times one of the patients wrote 'gk', which in the German language cannot be pronounced. Or else one finds the sound 'h' at a place where it is impossible to pronounce it. The patients ordinarily begin to write a word only after they have succeeded in pronouncing it. In writing they often repeat the word, sometimes aloud. Occasionally they speak correctly but write incorrectly. One of the patients once wrote 'Biln' instead of 'Berlin' although he had pronounced the word correctly.

Deformations of letters are as rare as deformations of sounds in ideokinetic aphasia. Beginning a wrong sound, be it in speaking or in writing, the patients notice the mistake, try to correct it, and the two intentions sometimes mix. In all incorrect letters we can perceive movements of the pencil in an attempt to correct the mistakes.

By virtue of the fact that the patients are able to write letters and numerals correctly, their capacity of copying properly can be explained. They also succeed in writing long words and sentences, because they separately copy the single letters. In the two male patients mentioned above slow writing and their constant movements of the eyes from the pattern to their sheet and back to the pattern could be observed. One of them wrote simple words such as 'die' and 'im' after one look at the pattern, but otherwise looked each time at the pattern before he wrote a letter; often he even looked several times before he wrote. The female patient acted differently. She wrote fluently and rarely looked at the pattern. In consequence her copying was just as incorrect as her writing to dictation. This patient, being a secretary, tried according to her habit, to survey whole sentences, and in consequence of her disorder could not do so adequately. Therefore, although trained in writing, she made more errors than the two unpractised patients, who only tried to do what they were able to carry out with the help of a pattern.

Thus, the writing disturbance of the patients corresponds to their speech disorder. They are able to speak as well as to write single sounds correctly, but they have difficulties in forming words, in speech as well as in writing. And in writing we also find the 'breaks' by which the speech is characterized. Whereas paragraphias are less frequent than paraphasias when the patients take pains to write correctly, the pauses last longer in writing than in speaking. Because letters follow one another more slowly than sounds, the patients are better able to stop in time so that usually the wrong letter does not appear. Frequently the patients must stop repeatedly and as a consequence the pauses are even longer. Often the patients bring their pencil near to the sheet and at once take it back again. These movements of the hand correspond to the slips in speaking. The patients intend to write a word, notice that it is incorrect, and stop.

Writing with the left hand does not produce mirror-writing. Indeed, writing with the left hand is occasionally more fluent than writing with the right hand. This is probably due to the fact that with practice, the right hand has grown independent of visual impressions, whereas writing with the left hand remains visually guided. An ideokinetic agraphia therefore affects left-hand writing to a lesser extent.

In conclusion, *ideokinetic apraxia, ideokinetic aphasia and ideokinetic agraphia all have the same kinesthetic basis. The single symptoms correspond entirely with one another.* Obviously the kinesthetic patterns for acting, speaking, and writing are disturbed. However, each of the three functions is so important for man that different areas in the brain are required. Clinical observations seem to confirm this. However, these areas are adjacent: *lesions of the parietal lobe produce an ideokinetic disorder of acting as well as of speaking and of writing.*

4. *Optokinetic agraphia and constructional apraxia resulting from ideokinetic apraxia for eye movements*

Luria (1966) registered the eye movements of patients while they were looking at pictures; he found severe disorders in case of lesions of the visual areas. Luria did not mention apraxia, but did mention incoordinate movements; perhaps, however, apraxic disturbances were involved. In describing the methods of investigation Luria notes that the patients were requested to look to the right or to the left, but he does not add whether they were allowed to move the head together with the eyes. This is decisive regarding apraxia, because patients suffering from apraxia for eye movements are able to move head and eyes to the side in a natural way. This is an action which occurs in every-day situations and the movement has been automatized, just as was described in ideokinetic apraxia of the limbs and of the face. However, when asked to keep the head immobile and to move only the eyes, the apraxic patient is unable to do so. Zutt (1932) described an 'apraxia of closing the eyes', but thought it was not a genuine apraxia but rather some other form of inability, presumably psychological. Waltz (1961) reported two cases of 'dyspraxia of gaze'. Seemingly the second case was characteristic of optokinetic apraxia. Mechrota, Anklesaria and Khosla (1964) described a congenital

44

'ocular motor apraxia'. Otherwise apraxia for eye movements is sometimes mentioned in connection with general facial apraxia.

Case No. 6. Anna Schen., born in 1908, a clerk, was suffering from severe constructional apraxia. She could draw or copy only the simplest figures. Copying was more impaired than spontaneous drawing; it was especially difficult for her to copy exactly some model. When requested to draw a square and then a triangle, she perseverated and drew a square twice. Her drawing of a key somewhat resembled a key, but when attempting to draw a heart, she produced a circle and then two ogives. Her drawing of a chair looked like a square angle. Asked to draw a house, she only drew a misshapen roof. When requested to copy a house, she did not really copy it, but drew a roof as before. The examiner had to name every part of the house so that she could draw it. The wall was first drawn beside the roof, and then under it. The windows were correctly placed but the door was drawn under the house. She did not pay any attention to the model, but only reacted to the requests which, because of her hesitations, had to be repeated over and over again. Really her drawings never resembled the models she was supposed to copy. Attempting to copy a cross, the patient failed and drew a square. When requested to copy a triangle, she added two sides to the model, so that it looked like a parallelogram. On repeated demand she first drew a square, then a triangle, not according to the pattern, but of a shape she had chosen herself. The same could be observed when she was to copy a square. She drew a rectangle, remarked, when questioned, that one dimension was too long, and succeeded in drawing a square, which, however, was too large in comparison with the model. Requested to correct her drawing, she only changed one dimension so that it became a rectangle again. She was unable to adapt her drawing to the model. It could also be observed that the model was not useful to her; she only hastily glanced at it and then looked perplexed to the side or toward the examiner. Finally she drew quickly and without paying attention to the model. A cross, which she could not draw on the sheet, was drawn by her with her hand correctly in the air, a circle also. However, she was unable to form more difficult figures in the air.

The constructional apraxia manifested itself in a like manner, or even more significantly, when the patient tried to shape figures with matches. Sometimes she formed a triangle correctly, but was unable to copy a square. One side was left open. She also was unable to put two matches in the shape of a 'T'. Instead she formed an angle. When asked what she thought of it, she said the letter was wrong, but she was not ready to correct it, stating that she was not able to do so. Sometimes she put the matches into the models and in this manner completed or enlarged the figures.

To dictation she wrote some letters correctly, but others could not be recognized at all. As for words, the patient could only write her name, but the first name was incorrect and the surname not always correct. In copying letters the patient was more successful. But here also slips happened. She did not copy slavishly, but wrote in her own manner. When asked to stick to the model, whe wrote again in her own way, or else she failed.

Reading was not disturbed. The patient also correctly read words out of a medical text, such as: 'Repetitorium', 'Kapfengerger' (name), 'Beschlüsse' (resolutions), 'Strickrodt' (name), 'Ober-apotheker' (dispensing chemist), 'Dräxel' (name). She pronounced 'Repetitorium' a little slowly, the other words quite fluently. Reading a text which she did not know she occasionally made a mistake, but probably not more frequently than any other person. She also understood a text which was suitable to her education and her practical knowledge. She read simple numbers correctly. She correctly spelled simple words such as 'Braten' (roast meat), 'Bank' (bench), 'Frau' (woman), 'Mann' (man). In more difficult words she left out some letters. However she was not able to form words with blocks on which letters were printed, even though she could spell these words correctly or pronounce them slowly while handling the blocks. She could tell whether a given word was right or wrong, but could not correct mistakes. She did not even try to do so earnestly, but after short attempts she looked in perplexed fashion to the side or toward the examiner. She turned over reversed letters.

She recognized and named objects correctly. She also recognized shapes which she could not draw. Because naming can only be examined with very simple forms, we examined the recognition of shapes in a different way. The patient was requested to put the 25 figures of Bernstein's memory test on outlines representing these figures. This she did properly, but she took more time than normal. In counting dots on a paper she made mistakes because she counted without order and forgot some dots and counted others twice.

Furthermore, the patient had a disorientation in space. In the hospital, during the first days, she had to ask the nurse where the toilet was and where her bed was. Later on she found both places by herself and in the examination room could adequately describe how to get to them. However, she failed entirely when she was asked to describe how to get to the city from her dwelling, be it on foot or by tram. She could not tell right from left. *Above* and *below* were correctly shown, but she made mistakes in distinguishing *in front of* from *behind.*

When the examiner drew stripes on her body with his finger she could not tell whether the direction was transversal or vertical. After some training the mistakes lessened. Asked to show where she was touched on the body she usually succeeded, but failed when not sufficiently attentive. She recognized numbers written on her body. Kinesthetic sensibility and stereognosis were intact. Recognition and naming of the fingers was greatly disturbed.

When examined for apraxia, the patient did not immediately produce correct movements with the right or with the left hand, but began rather to move uncertainly. Shown how to do it, she instantly imitated the movement correctly. Later she could also perform the movement on command. Movements of the face were all carried out correctly upon request, with the exception of the movements of the eyes. There was no apraxia of the eyelids; they could be opened and closed at will. The patient was also able to close the right and the left eye separately.

The fact that during examination for apraxia, the patient at first could not find the correct movements upon command, surely was due to her optokinetic defect, since stimulations from the visual sphere were missing. Ideokinetic apraxia can be excluded, because the patient from the outset could perform movements when shown how to.

In ideokinetic apraxia the imitation of the examiner's movements is impossible. This fact is not always taken into consideration in the literature. The patient was able to perform correct movements of the face upon command.

So far, the patient was suffering from pure agraphia without alexia, and from pure constructional apraxia, recognizing the figures she could not draw and being able to designate the mistakes she could not avoid. It is justified in this case of constructional apraxia to add *pure*, as no gnostic disturbances were involved. Since Kleist (1934) first described constructional apraxia several authors discussed whether this condition is a true apraxia or whether visuospatial perception is impaired (Duensing, 1953; Critchley, 1953; Zangwill, 1960; Gloning, 1965). Kleist separated 'Raumsinnstörung' from constructional apraxia and McFie and Zangwill (1960) distinguished it from visuospatial agnosia. Grünbaum (1930) and Lange (1936) treated the two disturbances as one entity called *apractognosia*.

In our patient we found in addition to constructional apraxia, disordered recognition of her fingers, confusion between right and left, and spatial disorientation, so that it may be surprising that I should speak of pure apraxia. But these symptoms are not decisive in this respect. *Pure* is an appropriate term for the apraxia in our patient because her praxic difficulties were not at all related to visual gnosia, for she recognized all her mistakes; she knew and named correctly all figures she could not draw; she could not form words from blocks on which letters were printed, but could show exactly where she had been mistaken.

Besides the constructional apraxia the patient was suffering from a severe apraxia for eye movements, though she had apraxia neither of the hands nor of the face. In spontaneous behaviour no disturbance of eye movements could be observed. She looked at the surrounding objects in a natural way, looked at the person to whom she spoke, turned aside when addressed from there, or when her attention was attracted from there in some way. So the disturbance could be overlooked, and surely was overlooked, by some examiners. However, when writing or drawing, our patient often looked in a direction different from that which she had to look to see the examiner or the model. She looked hastily at the model and then looked aside. This could be explained by her insight into her disability, but still it was astonishing that all encouragements and exhortations to look at the paper were often quite useless. As a matter of fact when requested to look aside, toward the window, or toward the door, the patient did so by turning her head and her eyes. She could also look upward and downward. But when asked to look only with her eyes, keeping the head immobile, she did not succeed at all. In each attempt she also moved her head. As long as she only tried to follow the request, the eyes often performed short movements in different directions. But as soon as significant movements set in, the head was involved. After a longer effort to follow a command, her eyes often did not move together with her head; sometimes her head was turned far aside while the eyes kept looking straight ahead. The glance of the patient was not attracted by the examiner. When he stood beside her, her eyes continued to be directed forward, while her head turned toward the examiner. In the same way she could not look upward or downward without moving her head, no matter whether the examiner stood in front of or beside her.

The same failure of the patient was to be observed when she was asked to look at the finger of the examiner, no matter whether the finger was first held at her midline and from here was moved in different directions, or whether it was from the beginning held up or down or beside the patient. In no case did the patient succeed when keeping her head motionless. Again only short movements in different directions followed. When her head was held fast, it vigorously tried to move where the eyes had to move. Only when the head was absolutely fixed did the eyes sometimes move alone as was desired. Usually they returned immediately. In this inability of the patient to follow the moving finger, there was no difference whether the examiner stood in front of her or beside her, whether in consequence the patient had to look at him or had to avert her eyes. Even if the examiner, while standing by the side, kept saying 'Look here! Look here!', the eyes, when the head was held fast, moved only transiently slightly in the desired direction. Optokinetic nystagmus was intact. It only lasted a short time while the patient was looking at the rotating drum.

In this manner apraxia for eye movements manifested itself. We have to assume an ideokinetic form of apraxia. As is generally characteristic of ideokinetic apraxia, the movements were correctly performed in natural situations, but were incorrectly performed when carried out upon command. So in the natural synkinesis of head and eyes the movements were adequate. In a general facial apraxia an apraxia for eye movements is also found. The patient suffering from a general facial apraxia sometimes also turns his head more than his eyes, but when his head is held fast, he will move the eyes alone. Perhaps the movements of the head become so obvious in isolated apraxia for eye movements because the head is not involved in the apraxic condition, whereas in general facial apraxia the head is apraxic also. The movements of the head were not the only mistakes of our patient. In attempts to move her eyes, there were slight movements in different directions, thus the eyes also derailed.

We must also consider the possibility that isolated apraxia for eye movements, though being ideokinetic, is a special form of apraxia with a special feature. At any rate it must have a special localization in the brain, since it can, as our patient demonstrates, appear without general facial apraxia. This form of apraxia seems to be of importance in the origin of agraphia and constructional apraxia. Probably an independent area in the brain is necessary to make writing and constructing possible.

Further, we might consider that the disorder observed in our patient is caused only by our separating eye movements from head movements, which are very closely associated normally. In most cases we simultaneously move head and eyes. But normal synkinesis does not compel us to do so. For instance, when we rest our head or our arm, in looking we only move our eyes. When watching from a place of concealment, we also purposely move only our eyes. There are many mimical eye movements in which the head is not involved (Leonhard, 1968). Referring to mimics we can even maintain that isolated eye movements are a very old ability of man. There is thus no reason to consider the phenomenon in our patient as being different from apraxia.

As a consequence an important question arises: Is there a relationship between agraphia and constructional apraxia and apraxia for eye movements? As we have seen, agraphia is also found in ideokinetic apraxia and ideokinetic aphasia. But in these cases the forming of letters was not disturbed but only the composition of words. In writing the forming of letters is obviously not dependent on the function of the hand. Indeed, though we learn writing only with the hand, usually the right hand, we are able to write with other parts of our body, especially with the left hand, with the legs, and even with the mouth. What is written via these other possibilities is extremely unskilled, rude, and messy, but the letters and words are principally written correctly so that we cannot speak of a true agraphia. It is quite unlikely that the different parts of the body learn to write and to draw with the help of the right hand. It is known that in writing with the right hand the symmetrical muscles of the left hand unconsciously participate in training, but in this way mirror writing arises, which is irrelevant here. We can also convince ourselves in writing with the foot or with the mouth that we are guided by the visual picture of the letters and words, not at all by thinking of the movements of the right hand. So it can be stated that we write and draw, so to speak, with the eyes, and only the finer shaping of the letters do we perform with the right hand. This statement may be a trifle surprising since with the eyes we cannot carry out writing movements in an arbitrary manner, because the eyes move by jerks and do not perform the curves of the letters. The jerks often make the movements pass the limits so that not even the general form of the letters is correct. But the eyes are able to follow a moving object exactly. Whereas we cannot freely describe a circle with the eyes, we can do so when looking at a rotating object, for instance at our own finger, describing a circle, or again looking at the point of a pencil moving. Surely we do this also when we learn writing, and in this way the eyes learn at the same time as the hand. Moreover, they learn more rapidly than the hand because the eyes, which embrace a much wider space, have more capacity regarding relations in space. While the hand still has to take pains, the eyes have full mastery and even are able to guide further training of the hand. They guide other parts of the body a well, when these try to write. It is not necessary for the eyes to be able to describe writing movements. It is enough that the movements which have been learned by following the point of the pen appear in mind. They do so not innervatorily but kinesthetically, and from this rationale we obtain confirmation that optokinetic agraphia is really not a motor but a sensory disturbance. On the other hand optokinetic agraphia is not a visual agraphia since visual knowledge is not disturbed, but rather kinesthetic knowledge.

Writing corresponds to drawing. This is likewise dependent upon the optokinetic function and so optokinetic apraxia corresponds to optokinetic agraphia. We must not think, however, that constructional apraxia is always optokinetic. It can also originate from a loss of gnosia. Then we have an apractognosia which corresponds to agraphia resulting from alexia.

The fact that people later write more rapidly and skilfully no longer refers to the eyes. Now the hand has grown somewhat independent and has in addition learned so much that the eyes are not able to learn. Regarding fine and rapid movements, the hand is superior to the eyes.

With these considerations we can really state that in our patient optokinetic apraxia resulted in an inability to write and to draw. The optokinetic patterns, i.e. the kinesthetic patterns of eye movements, which are necessary for writing and drawing, have been lost.

The only function preserved in our patient is that which is not dependent on the eyes; that which is due to the increasing skillfulness of the hand. She was not able at all to copy but wrote some letters in her individual handwriting. She was unable to write words, because visual control would be necessary, but she could sign, since signing in persons skilled in writing can be carried out automatically by the right hand. In drawing she succeeded in simple forms such as a circle or a cross, which also do not need visual control. Neither in writing nor in drawing could she copy anything.

In drawing the patient could not turn her movements in the direction she wanted because she no longer possessed the kinesthetic patterns of the eye movements. These patterns were also lacking when she was asked for directions in space, for direction to the right, to the left, within the ward, or regarding the streets of the city. Visual knowledge alone is not enough to determine the directions. Eye movements must help, through kinesthetic images. In consequence of her optokinetic apraxia the patient no longer knew directions. She could distinguish *above* from *below* or *front* from *back* because control by the eyes is not necessary when different parts of the body are concerned. But the right side and the left side of the body are symmetrical and the eye movements must help determine the direction. As regards knowledge of finger movements not only their shape is decisive, but also their succession in a certain direction. In other cases there may be visual agnosia, but in this case the difficulties were the consequence of the optokinetic disorder. Visual gnosia was not disturbed.

Though pure agraphia and pure constructional apraxia are in like manner dependent upon apraxia for eye movements, the two disorders may result from different lesions. Such important functions as writing and drawing probably require distinct, but adjoining, areas in the brain.

5. *Acalculia resulting from optokinetic apraxia*
In agraphic patients both a disturbance of calculation and a disorientation as to time have sometimes been found (Wernicke, 1903;

Erbslöh, 1903; Gerstmann, 1927; Liepmann, 1929; Zutt, 1932; Kleist [Fall Schnell], 1934). Sometimes impaired drawing is also mentioned, corresponding to the constructional apraxia later described by Kleist (1934). Contemporary authors are not so keen on describing pure cases so that it is difficult to decide whether these two symptoms – agraphia and apraxia on the one hand, disorders of calculation and orientation on the other hand – are more closely related to each other than are other symptoms. Hécaen, Angelergues and Houillier (1961) reported no fewer than 183 patients suffering from calculation disorders combined with very different symptoms. These authors set forth three categories of acalculia, depending upon whether the disturbance was found in the reading of numbers, or in arithmetical operations, or in the capacity for spatial organization in number notation.

Cases of acalculia without agraphia and constructional apraxia do not refute the assumption of a close relationship because there are different types of calculation (Leonhard, 1939 and 1940), and in consequence exceptions must occur. Some people perform elementary calculations automatically, i.e. from the sound of the numbers. Individuals in this category solve all elementary tasks the way other people solve simple multiplication tasks. For such persons ('Zahl-wortrechner') disorders are to be expected whenever there is a lesion in the auditory sphere. Another category of persons 'write in their minds' the figures they have to manipulate ('Zahlbildrechner'). Disorder of elementary calculation in these cases is combined with an agraphia for letters. A third group of persons shape in their minds diagrams by which they carry out their calculations. In cases of constructional apraxia they are no longer able to shape these diagrams, and acalculia follows. In the third category simple multiplications are solved automatically, but all other tasks with the help of mental diagrams. According to Spalding and Zangwill (1950) Galton was the first to mention these diagrams. Spalding and Zangwill took the diagrams into consideration in their study of acalculia, but did not describe them distinctly. Nor did they distinguish several types of calculation. Figure 1 shows the calculating diagrams of two physicians.

It has sometimes been maintained that calculations based on the multiplication tables are always performed purely from the sound of the numbers, but in fact, for the second category numbers are also

53

written in the mind for this kind of task. And this category out-numbers the other two. Of 91 healthy persons whom I could ask, 29 belonged to the first group, 41 to the second, and 21 to the third.

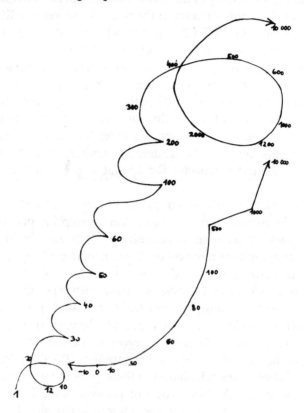

Figure 1. Calculation diagrams of two physicians.

Because there are different calculation types, the disorders of calculation are more differently localized in the brain than are other neuropsychological functions (Cohn, 1961; Critchley, 1953). A preservation of the multiplication tables can be expected only in the third type. In fact, Kleist (1934) in his cases found all calculation operations simultaneously disturbed. On the other hand exceptional cases confirm the existence of the third type. Poppelreuther (1917), Peritz (1918), Lange (1930), Bürger-Prinz (1935), and Lindqvist (1936) described patients in whom the simple multiplication tables were preserved. Berger (1926) described a patient who had lost only the multiplication tables. Because the lesion was found in the temporal lobe, the relationship to the auditory sphere was confirmed.

Schulze (1959) took into consideration the different types of calculation. He observed a patient who showed acalculia including the simple multiplication tables. Because the disorder was associated with ideokinetic aphasia, Schulze could demonstrate the relationship of acalculia to apraxic language. So the first type of calculation was assumed. In visual types of calculation we shall find a disturbance of visual praxia, i.e. an optokinetic apraxia, leading to an optokinetic agraphia.

Gloning (1965) in two cases could also distinguish different types of calculation. Both patients had a parieto-occipital tumor. In one patient with a severe calculation disorder, the simple multiplication tables were preserved, so that Gloning could assume that the patient used to calculate with diagrams. In the other case the disturbance of calculation was slight, in spite of the same location of the tumor, so that an auditory type could be supposed.

Anna Schen. who was described in the preceding chapter, could not indicate the year and guessed December instead of November. Asked for her age she hesitated, said 40, then 41, then correctly 46. She could not indicate the dates of World War I and World War II nor the birth dates of her children. The date of her own birthday she knew. Her replies changed when questions were asked in a different way. On the second day of her stay in the clinic, when asked what she had brought with her on admission, she named a dress, a scarf, and a piece of toilet soap. She could indicate the trade mark of the soap and indicated correctly that she had not used the soap very much. It was still possible to see the make 'Luxor'. She described adequately the toothpaste she had brought with her. She told us that she had brought along a narrow comb, not her own broad comb. She did not know whether her husband had given her this comb to bring with her. Further she mentioned the hairbrush and correctly named the colour of it. Later in the examination room she correctly described her bedside table with the drawer in the ward and did not forget the shelf space under the drawer. She also knew whether and by whom she had been visited. On the contrary she failed again when she was examined by means of Ziehen's memory test and Bernstein's memory test. Out of 29 figures only three were correctly designated.

Calculation was severely disturbed. The patient was unable to solve simple divisions. She multiplied small numbers instead of dividing them. Of subtractions scarcely any were solved. She correctly worked out $20-10$, but did not succeed with $6-3$, $10-6$, or $20-9$. Asked $9-3$ she guessed 8, then 7. When adding, she failed when the sum exceeded 10. So she could not sum up $6+7$ or $8+3$. Also some problems of less than 10 were not solved, such as $4+5$. Two identical numbers she could correctly sum only if the sum was less than 10; she did not solve $6+6$. No task of the compound multiplication table was solved. On the contrary the patient still had full mastery of the simple multiplication table. She also solved 7×9, 8×7, and 7×6, which are a little more difficult. Asked 4×4 first she persistently replied 8, but in a later examination correctly said 16. Some times the patient hesitated; if we repeated the question she answered correctly immediately.

She was able to count up and also counted correctly from 100 downward. After a ten, she attempted to pass on to the next ten and repeatedly had to be requested to consider the units also; then she also named the units.

Writing of simple numerals was intact. In larger numbers she each time confused the tens and the units. Instead of 854 she wrote 845; instead of 7,824 she wrote 7,842. So she wrote the single ciphers as they are spoken one after the other in the German language (54= vierundfünfzig). Requested to write 6,340 she left out the 0. In reading numbers she regularly first tried to read the single ciphers one after the other. Instructed how to do it properly, she read numbers of 3 figures but usually confused the tens and the units. Numbers of 4 figures she could not read. Instead of 7,893 she read 739. She thus left out one cipher and confused the ten and the unit. Asked which of two numbers was the higher, she guessed and frequently was wrong. For example, she judged 30 to be larger than 17, but thought 33 was larger than 98.

The severe acalculia explains the failure of the patient in reading and writing large numbers. Someone who is no longer able to sum up $5+2$ naturally can neither read nor write 7,893. It is even surprising that the patient sometimes could read numbers of 3 figures. Surely she wrote mechanically, i.e. by 'short cut' without understanding the meaning of the numbers, as she could not even say which of the two numbers 26 and 84 was larger.

The complete inability to operate with numbers also explains her disorientation in time. The fact that she was a little weak of memory was not decisive. As mentioned, the patient could name exactly the objects she had brought into the clinic, the make on the soap, and the comb the husband had given her. Her failure in Ziehen's test is a matter of course because the numbers had no meaning for her any longer. In Bernstein's test she could not succeed because in consequence of her severe optokinetic apraxia, described above, she could no longer visually delineate the shapes used in the test, in order to memorize them.

Before her illness Schen. had undoubtedly claculated by the third method mentioned above, for in the disturbance the simple multiplication tables were not involved. Individuals belonging to this category cannot even do the simplest arithmetical sums, for instance 9+8, unless they use mental diagrams. Only for the simple multiplication tables can they omit their diagrams. Divisions within the multiplication tables which leave no remainder can also be performed without diagrams, but the initial number which is to be divided must be sought for on the diagram.

Our patient undoubtedly had lost her ability to form her calculation diagram just as she had generally lost the ability to shape geometric figures. Her acalculia is therefore a direct consequence of her optokinetic apraxia.

Generally, people who calculate by means of diagrams also use diagrams for divisions of time, i.e. for the hours of the day, the days of the weeks and the months, the important events in their private lives and the dates in world history. These chronological diagrams sometimes resemble the diagram for calculation, and sometimes are quite different. In optokinetic apraxia none of these diagrams can be shaped. In consequence, together with the ability of calculating, the patients *lose the memory of dates they knew before.*

6. *Pure agraphia and pure constructional apraxia resulting from disconnection*

In pure agraphia, i.e. without alexia, the classical authors repeatedly discussed a disconnection of centres (Pick, 1898; Wernicke, 1903; Berger, 1911; Henschen, 1922). Later, this concept, in consequence of the integral and dynamic ideas, was rejected. When I (1952) in a case of pure agraphia and constructional apraxia suggested a disconnection, I was contradicted (Conrad, 1953). Since then a change has come about. After the publication of Geschwind and Kaplan (1962) the disconnection syndromes were reintroduced (Geschwind, 1965; Russel, 1963; Lhermitte and Beauvois, 1973; Konorski, 1970; Botez and Crighel, 1971).

The classical authors, assuming a disconnection in agraphia, thought of an interruption of the pathways from the visual sphere to Exner's centre in the frontal lobe, in which a motor writing centre had been presumed. Kleist, however, suggested a disconnection between the visual sphere of the occipital lobe and the kinesthetic sphere of the parietal lobe in constructional apraxia. The following case illustrates this latter form of disconnection.

Case No. 7. Elisabeth Hab., born in 1893, a factory worker, was suffering from an erysipelas in December, 1950. After the fever had cleared up, a paresis of the left arm was found. The disturbance was probably the result of an embolic or thrombotic affection. In January and February, 1951, a thorough examination took place.

Ideokinetic praxia of the right hand as well as of the face was completely unimpaired. However, there was a significant dyspraxia of the left hand. Threatening, beckoning, and knocking were performed inaccurately. In thumbing her nose the patient did not succeed at all. A slight paresis of the left arm could be noted.

The patient had no difficulty in reading. However, texts which she did not know were read slowly. Sometimes she confused similar words such as 'Aufgabe' and 'Auflage', but corrected herself when the mistake rendered the sentence nonsensical. She could summarize what she had read. Greek words such as 'Pentameter' or 'Polytropos' she read slowly, letter by letter. Spelling was correct in short words such as 'Tinte' (ink), 'Feder' (pencil), and 'Löffel' (spoon). She also succeeded in writing 'Tischtuch' (table-cloth). But she skipped over a letter in each of the words 'Kaufladen' (shop), 'Fussboden' (floor), and 'Handtuch' (towel). In forming a word by means of blocks on which letters were printed she, in consequence of her constructive disturbance, had difficulties in placing the blocks exactly side by side. But she did not form wrong words. She turned over reversed letters. Numbers which were not too long were read fluently but she could no longer form large numbers. Instead of 25657 she read 256–57, i.e. she divided the number into two.

There were never any gnosic disturbances. She also recognized large pictures which could not be taken in at a glance. Spatial perception was intact. She could also describe a part of the city she knew. There was no ideational apraxia, no right–left confusion. In designating her fingers the patient was only uncertain in the beginning.

Writing was severely disturbed. In the beginning the patient was not able to write one single letter. Nor could she write her name. And it was impossible for her to copy isolated letters. Four weeks later she nearly succeeded in writing letters to dictation, but not in copying them.

The writing of numbers was also impossible in the beginning. The patient improved within a short time, however. Three days later she could write all numerals below 10 to dictation, but was not able yet to copy them. Even the numerals she had just written could not be copied. Later she seemed to copy numerals, but in fact she read the number and then wrote it without looking at the model. Therefore, she could not heed the size of the model, although she tried to. Thus writing of letters and numbers could no longer be guided by visual presentations. On the contrary, the use of a model disturbed writing, whereas she was able to write spontaneously again.

Once the patient could write most numerals to dictation, she was asked to write with her left hand. At that time she was no longer significantly apraxic on the left. Only one figure was drawn correctly (1), all other figures were drawn mirror-wise (2–9). When the examiner pointed to a 6 which the patient had reversed, she said: 'What is this? I cannot read it myself. Is it a 6? It is reversed.' This answer indicates that the patient knew the numbers very well, and yet her writing was not directed by this knowledge.

Hab. was asked to form geometrical figures with matches. Here again a severe disturbance manifested itself. The patient was not able to shape the simplest figures such as a triangle or a square, nor even an angle. With great difficulty she once succeeded in forming the letter 'T' with two matches; another time she did not even succeed in this. But she always knew whether or not a figure was shaped correctly according to the model. In case there was only an insignificant mistake, such as an angle not being exactly closed, she would say: 'Not quite correct', and she would point to the mistake. When a figure was turned by 90 degrees she also stated the mistake. When the figure was turned by 180 degrees, she said: 'Correct, but not quite.' After the figure was turned, she said: 'Now it is quite correct.' She was requested to put the 25 figures used in Bernstein's memory test on the corresponding 25 drawings of the pattern. Though some figures resemble each other, she did not err. She was exhausted after some time, as it is really difficult to properly select all figures. She was allowed to quit after she had placed 12 figures correctly.

We could also see the patient's intact gnosia from the fact that she was never satisfied with a wrong shape, but worked until she had succeeded, or stopped, sighing: 'I cannot do it.' So there were no wrong solutions, no incorrect figures. When matches were placed as in Figure 2, and the patient was asked to remove a match so that the two figures would resemble each other, she immediately did so. Then she was requested to replace the incorrect match exactly where it had been before. This was extremely difficult for the patient. She moved the match at once to the proper location but could not place it correctly. She moved it uncertainly to and fro, turning it one way and another. After many hesitations the match finally was placed correctly. The patient heaved a sigh of relief as if after some hard work.

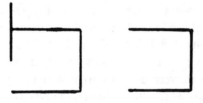

Figure 2.

Thus, Hab. knew the figures she could not shape. Moreover, she could match figures, did not fail to notice insignificant mistakes, and also differentiated figures which were turned. It is obvious therefore that she had no gnosic but only a praxic disorder.

This is again confirmed by the hesitating movements of the patient when working with matches. These were tentative movements by which the correct placement was sought. In observing the patient, when placing the matches uncertainly to and fro, we could see that she was not able to move them in the desired direction, but could move them only indiscriminately until by chance the correct position was found.

We encounter these tentative movements again in the drawing of

60

the patient. Such movements have also been reported by Seelert (1920) or by Lange (1930) but without comment. Liepmann (1900) stated that the pencil 'did no longer obey the intentions'. As for Lehmann-Facius (1951), he mentioned a 'hesitating seeking' in drawing.

Hab. failed in drawing just as in working with matches. Copying a triangle, she drew two sides more or less correctly, but the third side was completely erroneous. The patient, while drawing this side, shook her head angrily and showed that she had noticed the mistake very clearly. In a second attempt, because she was conscious of her inability, she drew one side and then made tentative movements, which, however, never took the direction she wanted. During these tentative movements, the point of the pencil repeatedly touched the paper, drawing a scatter of dots. There could be up to 26 tentative movements to the minute, which means that the patient again and again tried to find the correct direction.

After the patient had drawn the first line, she usually drew it again and again, instead of proceeding. And before drawing the first line, she regularly drew on the model. It was necessary to stop her repeatedly so that she did not destroy the model rather than copy it. Even though the pencil had been pushed away and the place had been shown again where she was to draw, she repeatedly drew on the model. Such closing-in could also be observed in writing and in shaping with matches. The model seemed to attract the patient like a magnet. Sometimes the examiner had to hold his hand protectingly beside the model of matches in order to keep it from being destroyed.

When drawing had somewhat improved, Hab. could draw better on request than when following models. On command she was now able to draw a square, a triangle, and a cross. Being requested to copy a triangle, she could not faithfully reproduce the model, and she knew it. Only at her fourth trial did she succeed in imitating the model somewhat better.

Just as was the case with writing, drawing could no longer be guided by visual impressions. Hab. could draw simple geometrical figures upon command, but could not draw them according to a model. However, she knew all the figures she could not draw, and when comparing different figures could state small differences between them. It would appear that a disconnection between the visual and the kinesthetic zone had occurred.

Hab. was also suffering from severe acalculia. She could not even make out $6+8$, $12-5$, 6×4, or $27+3$. She could only sum up and subtract numbers less than 10, and multiply and divide on the basis of simple multiplication tables. The disorder improved only slightly. Later on, she still failed in solving $34+13$, $24-7$, 8×8, and $48+8$. The calculation disorder also appeared in the reading and writing of larger numbers. Hab. was not able to form numbers with 5 digits, although she had no difficulties in reading the single numerals. When she could write single ciphers again, she could write multiple digit numbers more easily than read them. This supports the view that the disorder in the reading of numbers was the result of the calculation disability. In writing, the numbers can be composed without calculation, whereas in reading the position of the single numerals must first be decoded. Only units and tens are differently written and spoken in the German language.

Further, there was a disorientation as to time. January 3, 1951 she guessed to be February, 1913. She thought she was born in 1919. On the other hand, she knew that Christmas had occurred recently, and by this clue she identified the correct month. Regarding the last war, she knew the year 1944. First she thought the war began in 1933, then later she correctly cited 1939. Her temporal orientation improved, and six weeks later she knew the day of the month. About the events of her surroundings she always proved to be well informed. She failed in the memory tests of Ziehen and Bernstein.

Because she could no longer handle the multiplication tables, Hab. could not be considered a diagram user. She must have belonged to the visual calculation category. Calculation in the patient was dependent upon the reading and writing of numbers. Consequently the agraphia for numbers produced acalculia. When she later could write single ciphers, she surely did so mechanically, i.e. auditorily guided. But being a 'Zahlbildrechner' she needed the numbers presented visually and optokinetically. The dates of her personal life and of history are also founded on numbers and so were lost also. Perhaps Hab. was a little weak in memory, but this factor was not of great significance. She had not forgotten the events of which she could not recall the dates. She always knew whether she had been visited, or examined. She could tell details of the examinations. But she could never tell exactly at what time these events had occurred.

Why is a *disconnection* to be assumed in Hab., although this was not the case for Schen. (case No. 6), who showed a similar feature?

An important difference between Schen. and Hab. is that the two women were educated differently. Schen., who was a clerk, was much more trained in writing than Hab., who was a factory worker. That is why Schen., in spite of her agraphia, could write her name; she surely did so more or less automatically, whereas Hab. could not write anything at all.

In calculation the difference is due to the fact that Hab. belonged to a different calculation category than Schen. For Schen., calculation within the simple multiplication tables was preserved; in Hab. it was impaired. On the other hand, Hab. could write larger numbers than Schen.; after becoming able to write simple numerals again, she could compose 6 digit numbers, whereas Schen. usually failed even in 3 digit numbers. Schen. obviously no longer had any conception of numbers, for she thought 33 was higher than 98. Hab. was not asked such simple questions; surely she could have answered them correctly.

The acalculia was thus less severe in Hab. than in Schen. Is there any reason to assume that this lesser disorder was the result of a disconnection between the visual and kinesthetic areas, since in verbal calculation the hand is not involved? I have hypothesized that the 'Zahlbildrechner', who mentally write the numbers in their minds when calculating, do so only with the eyes, not with the hand, i.e. they act only optokinetically in their minds. But perhaps in ordinary people imaginary movements of the hand are helpful in calculation. We recall that the elements of calculation are learned by means of the fingers and that feeble-minded persons also continue to use their fingers in calculation.

Though belonging to different calculation categories, both patients were visually guided in calculating, whereas the patient of Schulze (1959), mentioned earlier, represented the auditory type, and in consequence had acalculia in connection with ideokinetic aphasia. This is also true for the second case of Richter (1962).

Again, Schen. was much more conscious than Hab. of what she knew and what she did not know. Very often she did not begin to act at all when requested, but declared that she was unable, or simply gazed perplexed straight ahead or at the examiner. Then she had to be urged again to try to perform the tasks. If she had shaped an incorrect form with the matches, she pointed at the mistake, but did not try to correct it. Asked to form words with blocks on which letters were printed, she failed in words she had spelled aloud correctly, indicated the mistake upon request, but here also did not attempt any correction. Though urged, she did not try to write with the left hand. Hab. behaved quite differently. She always seemed to be convinced of her ability to solve the task, for she regularly set out immediately to work and tried again and again. Only when exhausted after numerous fruitless attempts did she stop. Until then she obviously was of the opinion that ultimately she would succeed. The points on the paper produced by the tentative movements confirm the consistent attempts. Such behaviour was never found in Schen. She either acted or did not act, but she did not try to deduce the right movement.

Hab. was extremely inclined to write, to draw, and to put her hand into the model and to destroy it. Schen. moving incorrectly, occasionally would write on the model, but here it was definitely a slip. On the contrary Hab. seemed to be magnetically attracted by the model. The case reported by Zutt (1932) also drew on the model. This phenomenon of closing-in has been described by Mayer-Gross (1935), Critchley (1953), Ajuriaguerra and Hécaen (1960).

Hab.'s readiness to apply herself to the tasks can be explained by the fact that she always had in her mind the complete course of the desired movement, and so believed that she could immediately begin to act, whereas Schen. from the beginning hesitated as to the way she could perform the action. It is true that she was aware of the solution, for she was not agnostic, but she had no mental concept of the performing act. She had an apraxia for eye movements and could no longer determine the appropriate movements for writing and drawing. Praxia for eye movements was intact for Hab. so that in her mind she could act optokinetically. Since in spite of this the actual movement was incorrectly performed, a disconnection has to be assumed between the optokinetic zone and the ideokinetic zone of the arm, where the performance is to be arranged. The patient again and again started to move, but noticed that her arm moved differently from what she had in mind.

In Hab. we found not only a readiness to act, demonstrated by the closing in, but also a magnified inclination to apply herself to the tasks. In this connection, it is well to remember that the dependence

64

upon sensory impressions is a reflex action and as such is mediated through deeper pathways. Surely we are correct in supposing that the energy of acting, obstructed in its normal path, is turned aside to the deeper pathways. In the other patient, Schen., nothing was obstructed; therefore there was no occasion for deeper associations to be involved.

In order to verify the assumption of a disconnection syndrome in Hab., special examinations took place. To be sure, the exact opto-kinetic area could hardly be expected to be disconnected from the ideokinetic area for the arm. Probably the entire visual sphere was separated from the kinesthetic sphere. If this hypothesis is true then kinesthetic impressions can no longer be understood visually. This was found to be the case in Hab. Clinical examination failed to un-cover any disturbance of stereognosis. Hab. without hesitation named objects placed in her hand, with her eyes closed. Nevertheless she was unable to recognize numbers written with a finger on her skin. The numbers could be written on the right arm or the left arm, on the chest or on the leg, she recognized none of them. Even numbers drawn as large as the whole forearm were not identified. A cross drawn on the back of her hand was mistaken for a line. A very large cross drawn on the chest elicited the answer: 'Two lines.' Asked for the shape, the patient said: 'I don't know.' She did not recognize a circle either. Then she was told that she had only to distinguish between a cross and a circle. She now usually identified the stimulus correctly, though hesitatingly. When she had to indicate the direction of a line drawn on her skin, she could distinguish between upwards and downwards, but transverse lines were identified as upward or downward lines. After being informed that some lines were trans-verse, she hesitated when the next transverse line came and said: 'I don't know.'

After these results the sensibility was examined again. The patient noticed the slightest touch, on the right as well as the left side. She correctly named all objects placed in her hand, with her eyes shut. Kinesthetic sensibility in the right fingers and toes was entirely intact. Only for the left hand did mistakes sometimes occur.

Three months later the impairment in dermolexia was still pro-nounced. The patient did not recognize a cross drawn on the skin anywhere on her body. However, she now identified parallels correctly, even when drawn transversely.

Thus, there was a striking difference between stereognosis, which was intact, and dermolexia which was severely impaired over the whole body. This difference resulted from the fact that dermolexic stimulations had to be turned into visual concepts in order to be identified. And this the patient could not do. She could not recognize signs drawn on her skin because she could not form visual representations on the basis of tactile sensations. Thus, there was not only a disconnection which caused an inability to write and to draw. In addition, the kinesthetic-tactile sphere was severed from the visual sphere. To be more precise, both kinesthetic-tactile spheres, the right as well as the left, were disconnected from the left (dominant) visual sphere. The fact that Hab. recognized vertical lines better than horizontal is easily understood by the fact that *above* and *below* are more different on the body itself than *right* and *left* and so visual control is less necessary.

If this explanation is correct, stereognosis should be intact only for those objects which are quite familiar to the patient from tactile impression. With unfamiliar objects or with objects of unusual size, identification should be more difficult. Accordingly, the following objects from a doll's house were given to the patient, while she held her eyes closed. Since it was quickly discovered that what she did not recognize with the right hand she did not recognize with the left hand either, nor with both hands, she was allowed to use both her hands at the same time. The results were: *Bench:* 'Small board.' *Chair:* 'I don't know.' *Table:* 'This is wood.' *Frying-pan:* 'This is of sheet metal, I cannot name it.' *Spoon:* 'Small spoon.' *Clothes-peg:* 'This is an exceptional thing ... I don't know.' *Fork:* 'Hook ... something like a fork.' *Cup:* 'Lid ... or an inkstand ... a small vessel ... of enamel or metal.' *Ladle:* 'A piece of wood with a curvature in.' *Plate:* 'A small shell.' *Twirling-stick:* 'I don't know.' *Kitchen-knife:* 'Something of metal.' After this failure Hab. was informed that all objects had been taken from a doll's house. Now the result was: *Chair:* no response. *Bench:* no response. *Table:* 'This is a table or something like that.' *Clothes-peg:* (after prolonged touching): 'This is a peg.' *Frying-pan:* 'Spoon or something like that.' *Fork:* no response (though guessed correctly before). *Spoon:* no response (though guessed correctly before). *Cup:* 'Pot ... this is a handle ...' *Can:* 'Small cup or something like that.' *Kitchen-knife:* 'Of iron' ... no further response.

Then the objects were shown to the patient. Smilingly she confirmed that she knew all of them. She was then guided to the kitchen of the ward and, with her eyes shut, she named all kitchen-utensils correctly without hesitating.

So Hab. was not able to recognize objects by touching in case they were of unusual size, such as the implements of a doll's house. Through training, however, she could learn to recognize them by touching. When she was examined for the third time, she smilingly stated that these were the same small objects and named many more of them correctly than she had before. The results this time were: *Frying-pan*: 'Spoon.' *Bench*: 'Small chair.' *Cup*: 'Small pot.' *Can*: 'Also a small cup.' *Basin*: correct. *Clothes-peg*: correct. *Knife*: correct. *Ladle*: 'I don't know.' A healthy person easily recognizes the same objects even when touching them with only one hand.

These results are impressive and confirm the disconnection. They prove that tactile-kinesthetic impressions could not be translated into visual concepts. By sight, we get to know every object in different sizes, for as we come closer, an object grows larger, and each time we move away it becomes smaller. Therefore, a person who visually recognizes a large table will also recognize a small table. However, in the tactile-kinesthetic sphere, sizes remain constant; the impression of touch is always the same. Therefore, we learn to know the objects by tactile sense only in one size. When they are of unusual proportions, the impression must be translated into a visual image in order to be understood. In Hab. this was no longer possible, and consequently she could not identify the objects of the doll's house.

7. Origin of left-handed mirror writing

Some agraphic patients, when they try to write with the left hand, show mirror writing. The main reason why this is so is that in learning to write, stimulations from the left hemisphere are transmitted to the right hemisphere, where the corresponding movements are also trained to some extent. However, adductive (or abductive) movements of the right hand and adductive (or abductive) movements of the left hand go in opposite directions, so that when the left hand is used it writes mirror-wise. Similarly, according to Liepmann (1900), the left hand learns to unscrew when the right hand learns to screw. The dominant hemisphere can learn also from the minor hemisphere. A violinist having trained his left hand cannot play the violin well with the right hand, but assuredly his right hand is not as unskilled as the right hand of someone who has never learned to play the violin. Normally the training through transfer from the opposite hemisphere passes unnoticed. It is not necessary to suppose, as Pfeifer (1922) did, that the movements of the other hand are usually suppressed; on the contrary we must ask why a latent capability sometimes emerges in pathological conditions.

As was mentioned earlier, we learn to write optokinetically, i.e. under the guidance of eye movements, and in this manner we can also write with our foot or with our mouth. In case the optokinetic influence is lost, only the right hand can guide and it necessarily does so by stimulating the symmetrical muscles of the left hand. So mirror writing appears. *This finding always indicates that optokinetic guidance has been lost.* On the other hand, if agraphia is parallel to, and combined with, ideokinetic apraxia of the right hand, mirror writing is not observed.

To a certain degree we are usually able to neglect optokinetic guidance. We can, for example, write our names automatically because we have written them so very often. When trying to write the name with the left hand, without thinking and without hesitating, we involuntarily begin to use mirror writing.

The capacity to form mirror writing varies from individual to individual. Left handers, if they learn to write with the right hand, often have less difficulty in using mirror writing, because mirror writing depends on the right hemisphere, i.e. here the dominant and more capable hemisphere. Besides, in such a case the subordinate hemisphere (left) probably takes more time to learn, so that the dominant hemisphere can be trained longer. An observation of Bertha (1942/43) that mentally retarded people, when asked to write with the left hand, occasionally begin to use mirror writing, can also be explained in this way. The following case is an illustration of what has just been put forward.

Case No. 8. Elisabeth Bob., 53 years old. Since she was a baby she had not been able to move her right hand well. Later she attended a school for slow children because of the clumsiness of her right hand. She learned diligently and made progress. After completing school, she remained in the household of the parents.

Because of obsessional phenomena the patient was admitted to our

68

mental clinic in Berlin. In addition to a slight hemiparesis of the right arm and right leg, there was a considerable athetosis of the right arm.

As we began to examine her penmanship, she told us that she had been obliged at school, in spite of her handicap, to write with the right hand. This she managed to do but with great difficulty and only by means of an expedient. In order to eliminate the disturbing athetotic movements as far as possible, she used to fixate her hand with her cheek. Only in this manner was she able to direct the pencil adequately. Figure 3 shows the posture of the patient in writing.

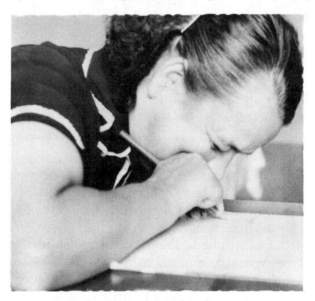

Figure 3. Posture of the patient in writing.

In the course of our dialogue the patient also told us that she could write much better with the left hand, but no one could read this writing, not even she. On request she wrote with the left hand and produced mirror writing. Figure 4 shows her usual handwriting (above) and what she wrote with the left hand (below). When one looks at the latter in a mirror one can see that it is much neater than the normal handwriting produced by the right hand, in which the letters are consistently misshaped by the athetotic movements.

Perhaps the obsessional phenomena from which the patient was suffering were not insignificant in regard to her writing. She was of

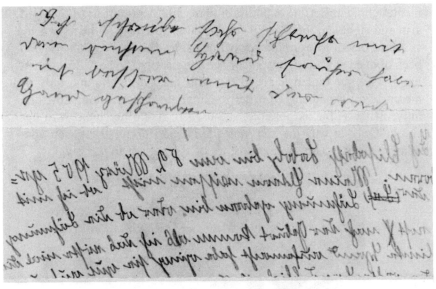

Figure 4. Right-handed writing and left-handed mirror-writing.

an anankastic nature and therefore was not only prone to obsessional ideas but also anxious to perform her duties to perfection. Probably for this reason she undertook the extremely hard task of learning to write with her athetotic hand.

The perfect handwriting of the left hand, which had never been trained, is the consequence of the right hand having learned much more intensively and for a much longer time than usual. When the left hemisphere at last had learned to write in spite of the athetotic movements, the right hemisphere, permanently stimulated from the other side, had also learned to write nicely. But only mirror writing had developed.

We now understand why mentally retarded people sometimes begin to use mirror writing. Surely some of them had great difficulty learning to write. Like our patient, they had to practice longer and more intensively than normal persons, so that the left hand had the opportunity to learn also. In left handers who incline to mirror writing, we must think not only of the better skill of their left hand, but also of the fact that in many cases, they had to laboriously learn to write with their right hand, i.e. with their subordinate left hemisphere.

70

That one hemisphere should benefit from what the other hemisphere learns to do is probably due to the fact that in grasping and catching with both hands symmetrical muscles must cooperate. As the right hand in many people is used much more frequently, the left hand in bimanual tasks would be very clumsy if it could not, to some extent, benefit from the practice the right hand has received. So, for example, it would not be possible to catch a ball by rapid grasping of both hands unless symmetrical muscles work together. Such co-operation reveals the training of both cerebral hemispheres.

8. *Pure agraphia resulting from a lesion of the right hemisphere*

Why does pure agraphia so often result from a lesion of the right hemisphere? I am not thinking here of patients who are agraphic only in one hand, such as the 'Regierungsrat' described by Liepmann (1900). I am referring to cases who are agraphic with the right as well as with the left hand. Many such patients with a right hemispheric lesion have been observed. Reichardt (1918) in his case admitted a lesion in the right hemisphere. Herrmann and Pötzl (1926) referred to 7 cases and added 3 further cases, whose clinical features were less pure, but who also had lesions of the right brain. Later, cases were described by Zutt (1932), Kleist (the case Schnell, 1934), Duvoir and Bertrand (1935), Leonhard (1952), Critchley (1953), Piercy, Hécaen and Ajuriaguerra (1960), Dubois, Hécaen and Marcie (1969), Poeck and Kerschensteiner (1971), Heilman, Coyle, Gonyea and Geschwind (1973). Not all of these patients were left-handed. Hermann and Pötzl (1926) conclude from their observations that bilaterality of the writing centres seemed to be much more frequent than bilaterality of speech.

This conclusion is extremely astonishing, because writing is the function which in adult Europeans, almost without any exception, is performed with the right hand; left-handers in most European countries until recently were obliged to learn to write with the right hand. If there is a function for which localization in the left hemisphere could be regularly assumed (independent of handedness), then it is writing. Yet in agraphics we find many cases with the lesion on the right side. There is little relationship of speaking to other motor acts, so it would not be astonishing if speaking were often represented in the right hemisphere and motricity in the left, but it is quite incomprehensible that people who write with the right hand should have their writing centre on the right side, even though they are right-handers.

However, in most of the cases with right-sided lesions, temporary aphasic or alexic symptoms were also found, which, on the one hand, did not seem to be very important but, on the other hand, demonstrated that speaking and reading in these patients were also represented in the right hemisphere. This is also true of the cases published earlier when, as far as possible, pure cases were chosen. The patients of Potts (1901) and of Stier (1917) quoted by Herrmann and Pötzl (1926) had both aphasic and alexic symptoms. But these patients were left-handed. The patient of Seiler (1914) and the second patient of Pelz (1913) were also left-handed. The first patient of Pelz had motor and amnestic aphasic disturbances, the second had amnestic aphasic problems. The patient of Semi Meyer (1908) and also the patient of Herrmann and Pötzl (1926) showed amnestic aphasic symptoms. The patient of Lewandowsky (1911) had sensory aphasic disorders, just as did the patient of Duvoir and Bertrand (1935). The patient of Zutt (1932) had alexic disorders in the beginning. Kleist's (1934) patient, Schnell, showed a transitory loss of speech.

Thus the question is somewhat complex. It can be assumed that patients who become agraphic after damage to the right hemisphere have a right-sided representation of speech and of reading, even though they are not left-handed. As a matter of fact, Marinesco, Grigoresco and Axente (1938) reported several patients for whom, in spite of right-handedness, a lesion in the right hemisphere was associated with aphasia. The same is true of a patient of Schaechter (1935). Conrad (1932/33) dealt with the problem statistically and found 5.8% of right-handed aphasic patients with lesions in the right hemisphere. So in a small number of patients we can expect the right hemisphere to be linguistically dominant in spite of right-handedness. However, more frequently, we find the reverse, left-handed persons with a dominant left hemisphere (Hécaen and Angelergues 1962). In left-handed patients, linguistic dominance is not so pronounced as in right-handed patients, so that recovery from aphasia is usually more complete (Quadfasel, 1954; Subirana, 1958; Zangwill, 1960; Botez and Calcaianu, 1961; Anastasopoulos and Kokkini, 1962; Hécaen and Ajuriaguerra, 1963). Agraphic patients with lesions in the right hemisphere seem to belong to the small number of individuals in whom language is represented in the right hemisphere, regardless of handedness. In spite of the right hemisphere being dominant for speech, it would be astonishing if writing was also represented in the right hemisphere, since even in these cases motricity is surely guided by the left hemisphere if there is right-handedness. I cannot concur with the explanation of Herrmann and Pötzl (1926) or of modern authors such as Piercy and Smyth (1962) that writing might be more frequently represented in the right hemisphere than other neuropsychological functions.

Let us return to the fact that writing in Europeans is learned and performed with the right hand. When the left hand is trained, mirror writing results. From this it can be concluded that writing is always represented in the left hemisphere. We could hardly imagine that in some people writing would be learned in the right hemisphere and from there transmitted to the left hemisphere; and that the right hemisphere would be involved again if mirror writing was observed. The right hemisphere would then have two centres, one for normal writing, one for mirror writing. This is extremely unlikely. Even in left-handed persons writing is certainly represented in the left hemisphere if writing has been learned with the right hand. At first it seems even less understandable that writing disorders should so often be associated with damage to the right hemisphere. However, the notion of disconnection enables one to account for this.

In Hab. (case No. 7) it could be shown by clinical analysis that the graphic and constructional apraxic disturbance was produced by interruption of cortical pathways. This disconnection can occur more easily if there is a longer route between the regions which must be interconnected. If there are persons in whom reading is learned in one hemisphere and writing in the other, then a lesion in the white matter frequently may involve the connection, for the pathways here run through the corpus callosum. In spite of Liepmann's impressive case, the significance of this part of the brain for agraphia and apraxia was denied for a long time. In recent years, however, the observation of Liepmann (1900) was confirmed (Geschwind and Kaplan, 1962; Gazzaniga, 1962; Geschwind, 1965; Gazzaniga, Bogen and Sperry, 1967). Lhermitte and Beauvois (1973) emphasize that the corpus callosum was too long neglected in this respect.

Interruption of long pathways through the corpus callosum must have occurred in cases where agraphia is associated with a lesion of the right cerebral hemisphere. The accompanying aphasic and alexic disorders, partly also the left-handedness, indicate that speech and reading are represented in the right hemisphere. Nevertheless writing is, as was pointed out, dependent on the left hemisphere. So, in these cases the connection between the two important regions runs through the corpus callosum and can much more easily be disturbed than when the regions for speech and reading are in the same hemisphere as the region for writing. In the latter case a disconnection is also possible, though the regions are adjacent here. On the other hand, when the linking fibres travel a long distance, the disconnection can occur not only in the corpus collosum but also in the white matter of the right or of the left hemisphere. So we conclude that pure agraphias associated with left hemispheric lesions are also possible in persons for whom the phasic and lexic functions are represented in the right hemisphere.

In cases of a commissural disconnection we expect apraxia of the left hand corresponding to the case of Liepmann. This is also confirmed by our patient Hab., for she showed a slight ideokinetic apraxia of the left hand, whereas the right hand remained free of involvement. The same is true of other cases of pure agraphia. The second case of Pelz (1913) had an ideokinetic apraxia of the left arm. The patient of Zutt (1932) had apraxic disorders, on the left side more than on the right in the beginning. The patient of Boettiger (1922) neglected the left arm, did not use it spontaneously, though there was no motor disorder. The same is reported by Herrmann and Pötzl (1926) regarding their case. So there are several patients confirming the notion of disconnection. More impressive would be an anatomical confirmation. The patient of Geschwind and Kaplan (1962) in whom the destruction of the corpus callosum was confirmed had agraphia only with the left hand so that he is not relevant here. The patient of Seiler (1914) had a malacia in the right hemisphere, which involved the largest part of the supramarginal gyrus, a part of the angular gyrus and a small field of the postcentral gyrus. The involvement of the white matter is not clearly described, but possibly the pathways from the parieto-occipital region to the corpus callosum were interrupted. Berger (1911) answers the question himself whether agraphia was produced by damage to the cortex or to the white matter: 'Lesions in the cortex are not to be found.' He concludes: 'The case shows that by interruption of nerve fibres alone such disorders of writing can arise.' In the patient of Kleist (1934) the lesion of the right hemisphere involved predominantly the white matter. The case of Berger particularly supports the concept of a disconnection in pure agraphia.

Several classical authorities suggested an interruption of pathways (Wernicke, 1903; Pick, 1898; Berger, 1911), but they conceived only interruption of the pathways to Exner's motor centre in the frontal lobe. I think my concept, which is a different opinion, is confirmed by my examinations. The disorder in tactile recognition, shown especially by the difficulty in identifying objects from the doll's house, would not have arisen, if only the motor area had been disconnected from the visual area.

However, one fact is not yet clearly explained. Some of the cases which have been published are not quite similar to mine. In most of them, only spontaneous writing was impossible, but copying preserved. Also, these patients did not have the involvements in figure construction which I have seen. These patients could copy simple figures. My patient, on the contrary, failed even when attempting to copy in exact fashion.

In German literature the two forms of difficulty can be well separated. Copying was less disturbed in the patients of Pick (1898), Byschowski (1901), Wernicke (1903), Erbslöh (1903), Berger (1911), Pelz (1912, 1913), Herrmann and Pötzl (1926), Gerstmann (1927), and Seiler (1914). Pelz and Gerstmann described two such cases each. The patient of F. Stockert (1942) also had other symptoms and copying was less disturbed. In other cases as in mine, copying was more involved than spontaneous writing. This is true for the patients of S. Meyer (1908), Kramer (1917), Boettiger (1922), Zutt (1932), two patients of Kleist (1934), namely Schnell and Otto, and the patient of Lange (1930), who, however, also suffered from other symptoms.

Surely there are essential differences between the two groups. It seems that in those cases which were more severely disturbed, the lesion was bilateral. In the patient of Boettiger (1922), a projectile had penetrated both hemispheres. The same is true for Kleist's patient Otto. In Kleist's patient Schnell, a traumatic lesion of the left hemisphere was complicated by a vascular lesion of the right hemisphere. The patient of Zutt (1932) had neurological symptoms from the right as well as from the left hemisphere. In my own patient, a lesion in both hemispheres must be assumed. In addition to the symptoms mentioned above, she also, in the beginning, had evidenced no reflex

75

movements of the eyes to the left nor to the right, and this can only be caused by a bilateral lesion. The patient of Kramer (1917) had the same disturbance as my patient and had earlier suffered from an apoplectic fit (cerebral lues). Out of the 7 cases mentioned, only the patient of Meyer (1908) showed no evidence of a bilateral lesion. However, prior to the apoplexy in Meyer's patient there were several attacks of dizziness and headache, perhaps resulting from slight apoplectic fits. The patient of Berger (1911) had bilateral damage, the second patient of Gerstmann (1927) initially suffered from a slight disturbance of tactile gnosis on the left side and paresis on the right side. The patient of Wernicke (1903) had several apoplectic fits earlier so that we can consider the possibility of bilateral damage. In other cases, no signs of a bilateral lesion have been reported. So in addition to these three cases, eight cases of the second group (those with copying less disturbed) remain, since Pelz and Gerstmann each published two case studies.

In fact, the findings indicate that the first group differs from the second by a bilaterality of the lesion. This is also confirmed by the fewer number of cases in the first group. Herrmann and Pötzl (1926) thought of a similar explanation, but objected to this opinion themselves, quoting information regarding the patient of Berger. However, if a lesion is bilateral, as in this case, it is not necessary that it should involve the regions important for writing in both hemispheres.

Indeed bilaterality of the lesion best explains the severity of the disturbance in our case and similar cases. Copying a triangle or writing a simple letter is surely not dependent upon the function of the dominant hemisphere. This task can also be subserved by the subordinate hemisphere. The fact that in cases of bilateral lesions spontaneous writing is not as severely disturbed as copying is also understandable, for the stimulations from the speech area, which are of no assistance in copying, can be helpful in spontaneous writing.

9. Conclusions

Our knowledge of aphasia has enormously improved since the time when, more than 100 years ago, Broca described the features of motor aphasia, and Wernicke the features of sensory aphasia. However, the authors did not reach a uniform scientific view. Now as ever opinions differ as to whether there are specific types of aphasia which can be related to lesions in certain regions of the brain. In the present monograph we have tried to demonstrate by decisive observations that there exists a language disorder with a well-defined picture that corresponds to a certain type of apraxia. The language disturbance as well as the apraxia are to be related to the parietal lobe which in contrast to the temporal lobe and frontal lobe, has been too much neglected as far as aphasia is concerned. In this monograph ideo-kinetic aphasia (parietal aphasia) is described in connection with ideokinetic apraxia (parietal apraxia). Further disturbances are identified as ideokinetic, namely a certain type of agraphia and a certain type of acalculia. Concerning other types of agraphia and of constructional apraxia, we had to refer to disconnection syndromes which, once described by Wernicke and Liepmann, are again widely taken into consideration by modern authors. It is hoped that the clinical cases reported here may help solve the complicated problems that still face aphasiologists.

2

PURE WORD BLINDNESS:
AN OVERVIEW

YVAN LEBRUN, RICHARD HOOPS, GUY MONSEU,
ANDREA COLLIER, NICOLAS STOUPEL

On October 17th, 1906, the French journal *La Semaine Médicale* published a polemic paper in which the author, Pierre Marie, denied the possibility of there being a selective impairment of oral language comprehension following brain damage. Rejecting classical teachings, Marie contended that pure word deafness was a myth. 'A mon avis,' he wrote, 'la surdité verbale pure est une forme d'aphasie absolument schématique et artificielle, sans existence réelle ni au point de vue clinique, ni au point de vue anatomo-pathologique.'

While he asserted that there was no such thing as pure word deafness, Marie conceded that there were patients with pure word blindness: 'Les faits cliniques démontrent bien que certains malades présentent un trouble de la lecture, sinon toujours absolument isolé, du moins nettement prédominant.'

As a matter of fact, Jules Dejerine, who was Marie's main opponent, had as early as 1892 given a masterly description of pure word blindness. Iconoclast though he was, Marie could not cast doubt on the reality of this selective impairment of written language comprehension.

The following three cases are typical instances of the syndrome of pure word blindness, also called pure alexia, optic alexia, visual asymbolia or agnosic alexia (Alajouanine, 1968, p. 125).

Case No. 1. In September 1976 a 72 year old right-handed man was referred by an ophthalmologist for neurological examination. For six months this French-speaking patient had had reading difficulties and right visual field defects.

By profession, he was a journalist and a painter. He had always been healthy apart from a brief and unique episode of syncope in 1974. Increased blood pressure (systolic pressure between 150 and 200 mm Hg) had been recorded for the past two years but no treatment had been prescribed.

One morning in June 1976, the patient noticed that objects around him seemed to be shining and that he had become completely alexic. After two weeks he recovered the ability to identify letters but not words. He could write but was incapable of reading over what he had been writing. He furthermore noticed some loss of peripheral vision to the right. There was no motor weakness, no sensory loss, and no speech disorder.

Despite his visual deficit he continued to paint, but his wife observed that his paintings had a slightly greyish appearance. The choice of colours was quite normal, however.

On neurological examination in September 1976, blood pressure was found to be 200/90. The heart appeared normal and no murmur could be heard in the neck. General physical examination was unremarkable. Cranial nerves were normal. There was no motor weakness, no sensory deficit (in particular, stereognosis and graphesthesia were normal) and no perceptual rivalry. Reflexes were normal and symmetrical. There was a right superior homonymous quadranopia.

The patient was conversant with current events and his general orientation in time was normal. However, he was mistaken when he had to say his age or that of his daughter.

He knew his address, but could not draw a map of his district nor find his way on a street map. There was no right–left confusion.

He had occasional difficulty in finding words, especially proper names, and in recalling dates of recent events.

He was verbose but did not use paraphasias. He could name objects on confrontation and he correctly answered even complex questions.

He could identify most isolated letters, but evidenced a slight tendency to perseveration. He could only read a few words and when shown a written sentence tended to guess at the constituents. Short words could be identified by sounding the letters one by one.

Telling the time was not always accurate. The reading of numbers was impaired and the patient was unable to dial a phone number. Mental as well as written calculation was disturbed.

Spontaneous writing and writing under dictation were fluent, with occasional omissions or doublings of words, letters or strokes. Most accents were either omitted or misplaced and the *t*'s were not crossed. The patient was unable to read over what he had written.

Spelling aloud from memory was impaired (it should be remembered that the patient used to work as a journalist and to type his papers himself).

The patient was unable to copy more than just a few words.

Although he used colours appropriately in his paintings, he could not name them properly, calling green 'violet' and pink 'orange'. However, he insisted that his verbal identification of colours was correct. He could match colours properly, even when subtle shades were used.

There was no finger agnosia, no constructional, ideomotor or ideational apraxia, no apraxia for dressing and no prosopagnosia.

There was no disturbance of personal body schema but the patient had recently been observed misplacing the big toes in a human figure drawn from memory.

Chest and skull X-rays were normal.

EEG showed theta and a few delta slow components over the left posterior temporal and occipital region.

CAT scan revealed an oval-shaped area of decreased density in the left occipital and posterior parietal convolutions. This hypodense zone was most probably an infarction resulting from a cerebro-vascular accident in the territory of the posterior cerebral artery.

Case No. 2. The second patient was a 62 year old French-speaking male who had been on medication for three years because of arterial hypertension and for 18 years because of diabetes mellitus. His mother had also been diabetic; she died of a cerebral thrombosis at 47 years of age. His maternal grandmother also had diabetes.

The patient was right-handed.

In April 1974 and again in June 1976 he had two spells of transitory aphasia.

In December 1976, upon awakening from a noon nap, he discovered that he had right hemiparesis (which he himself called *numbness*) and hypoesthesia, a visual field disturbance, and speech disorders.

The patient was admitted to the hospital and found to have total superior and relative inferior homonymous quadranopia on the right side. There was a right hypoesthesia for touch and pin-prick. Muscle strength was normal on either side. Tendon reflexes were present and symmetrical. Plantar responses were in flexion.

Comprehension of everyday conversation was normal but reaction time to requests indicated that the patient was slightly bradypsychic. Short-term memory was obviously disturbed, which rendered comprehension of stories difficult. Designation of fingers named by the examiner was faulty.

There was a moderate anomia especially for proper nouns. Occasional circumlocutions and paraphasias were noted.

Isolated letters and short words (such as articles, prepositions and pronouns) could be identified. Longer words were difficult to read. Sometimes the patient tried to identify them by sounding their letters one by one.

In the reading of sentences there were many morphological paralexias (*fils* was misread as 'fille', *lectures* was misread as 'lettres'). Paralexias were occasionally perseverative.

Handwritten sentences were much more difficult to read than printed sentences.

The patient could spell words aloud from memory and identify words spelled aloud to him.

Spontaneous writing and writing under dictation were correct, but the patient could not read over what he had written. Moreover, the right extremity of his lines was slanted downwards and was less legible.

Copying was extremely laborious.

Isolated figures could be easily read, but the reading of numbers was often erroneous. Mental and written calculation were moderately disturbed.

The patient could read the clock and dial telephone numbers. He could not remember them, however. He could not remember postal numbers either.

The identification of road signs was impaired, while geometric forms were correctly named.

Naming of colours on confrontation was faulty. This disorder cleared up relatively quickly.

The patient could no longer use a street map or explain a route in his native town. There was no left–right confusion.

Clinical investigation revealed a moderate renal insufficiency (creatininemia was 1.5 mg% with a clearance of 43 ml/min), without albuminuria.

Motor conduction velocity was 31.5 m/sec in the right common peroneal nerve and 51 m/sec in the right median nerve.

Left carotid arteriogram revealed a slight stenosis at the origin of the internal carotid artery and severe atheromatous lesions in the carotid siphon.

Vertebral arteriography showed atheromatosis of the upper half of the left vertebral artery with unwinding at the junction of the two vertebral arteries with the basilar artery. There was an atheromatous stenosis in the first segment of the right superior cerebellar artery and a total obliteration of the distal occipital and temporal branches of the left posterior cerebral artery (Fig. 1).

Case No. 3. The third patient was also a right-handed, French-speaking male. For ten years he had had arterial hypertension. In December 1968 – he was then 44 years old – he suffered an ictus which left him with a right hemiparesis, an important reduction of somaesthesia on the right side, an astereognosis of the right hand, an optocinetic nystagmus, a right superior homonymous quadranopia, a severe impairment of short-term memory and a fluctuating attention.

There was no finger agnosia, no right–left confusion, no spatial disorientation, and no facial paresis.

The patient had no difficulty in understanding spoken language and his own speech was fluent and correct.

On the other hand, owing to his important impairment of immediate recall, he was unable to reproduce a simple story he had just been told or to circumstantially answer questions about this story.

The patient recognized letters for what they are: being shown a card on which various signs (letters, figures, and non-alphabetic symbols) had been drawn, he was able to discriminate between the alphabetic and non-alphabetic signs. He found it difficult, however, to identify the individual letters: on one occasion, *H* was read as *N*, then as *H*; *O* was read as *K*, then as zero; *Z* and *F* were read correctly; *G* was read as *K*, then as *Q*; *Q* was read as *K*, then as *Q*; *U* was read as *U*, then as *V*; *T* and *V* were read correctly; and *B* was read as *F*, then as *P*, and finally as *B*. As may be seen, the mistakes were often due to confusion of letters of similar shape (H/N, U/V, B/F/P) or of similar sound (Q/K).

The patient found it even more difficult to read words. In order to tide over, he would sometimes guess. When shown the words *chateau*

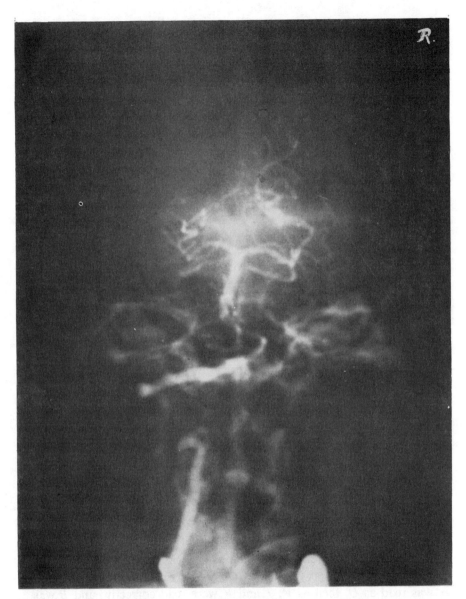

Figure 1

and *chapeau* and the image of a mansion, he misread *chapeau* as *maison*; when shown the words *chou* and *clou* and the image of a cabbage, he misread *clou* as *chou*.

84

When he could not guess at the word, the patient would usually try to identify the letters one by one and then to reconstruct the word. This procedure was all the more awkward as he was apt to forget the letters he had just been deciphering.

Sometimes the two methods were combined: the patient would identify the first letters of the word and then guess at the rest. On one occasion, the beginning of *parapluie* was spelt aloud *FA*, then *PA*, then the first syllable was read as *pa* and the whole word as *paraffine*. After a new inspection, the word was read correctly.

If the patient succeeded in identifying each word in a sentence and in remembering what he had identified, he could understand the sentence.

As a rule, figures were read more easily than letters, and numbers more easily than words.

On the other hand, the patient had no difficulty in writing either spontaneously or to dictation, but he could hardly read over what he had written once the memory of it had ceased to operate.

His handwriting was wide and clumsy: because of his right paresis he could not hold his pencil firmly and there was some degree of ataxia due to his impairment of somaesthesia.

He could spell words from memory and he could recognize words that were spelled aloud to him.

Provided he succeeded in identifying all the letters in a written word, he could generally tell whether the word had been written correctly or not.

He could solve anagrams provided he could find out and remember long enough which letters he had been given.

He was able to solve simple problems in addition, subtraction, multiplication and division, as long as he did not misread his figures.

Copying print into script was arduous because of his difficulty in reading.

Carotid arteriography showed the obliteration of the posterior temporal branch of the middle cerebral artery. No vertebral arteriography was done.

The three cases reported above very much resemble each other. A survey of published cases of pure word blindness reveals, however, that the syndrome may show considerable variation as regards the severity of the reading impairment, the kind of written material that can no longer be deciphered and the concomitant neurological or neuropsychological deficits.

Many pure alexics, including our three patients, find it more difficult to read words and sentences than letters. Their alexia is predominantly verbal. In some cases, it is exclusively verbal, the identification of individual letters remaining easy (e.g. Ajax's first patient, 1967). A few alexics, however, read words more easily than letters. Their alexia is primarily literal. In some of these cases (e.g. patient Bla. in Dubois-Charlier, 1971) the identification of individual letters is nearly always erroneous, while the reading of isolated words is moderately disturbed and the understanding of sentences but slightly impaired.

Some patients can recognize neither letters nor words. Comprehension of written language is completely blocked. Such patients have global alexia (e.g. Dejerine, 1892; Péron and Goutner, 1944).

Patients with pure alexia may find print easier to read than handwriting (e.g. our case No. 2; Hinshelwood's second case, 1902). Benson and Geschwind's statement (1969) that 'the most striking symptom recorded (in cases of pure alexia) is of course the inability to read printed material' is therefore misleading.

Some patients have less difficulty identifying isolated letters than letters in words (e.g. Stachowiak and Poeck, 1976). It is as if the simultaneous presentation of several letters made their individual identification more difficult. When he had to read a series of letters, Holmes' patient (1950) would complain: 'I don't know what letter I am trying to see.'

Patients with literal alexia often confuse letters which look alike (cfr. our third case; Ombredane, 1944, p. 110) or which sound alike (our third case).

Patients with predominantly verbal alexia not infrequently try to read words by sounding the letters one by one, i.e. working from the individual letters they reconstruct the sound pattern of the word in order to find its meaning. This makeshift is sometimes called *spelling dyslexia*.

Letters or words seen every day or in familiar contexts are usually easier to read. Although he was severely alexic, Warrington and Zangwill's patient (1957) could read the names of some daily papers and some popular brands of cigarettes.

Verbal alexics sometimes succeed in discovering the semantic field a given word belongs to, although they fail to identify the word itself. It is as if they could retrieve only part of the word's conventional meaning.

Conversely, when they know to which semantic field a word belongs, some patients can read it more readily. Beringer and Stein (1930) have described a patient who could not read lists of conceptually related words as long as she did not know to what semantic category the words belonged. As soon as she was told that the words she was to read denoted, say, tools, she could recognize most of them.

Semantic and morphological paralexias are frequent in patients who are not totally alexic. A patient makes a semantic paralexia when he mistakes a given word for a conceptually related word. For instance, Beringer and Stein's German-speaking patient (1930) once misread *Indien* (India) as *Elefant* (elephant). She spontaneously explained that she had immediately realized that the word referred to something exotic, something tropical. Then it dawned on her that the word must denote elephants.

In morphological paralexias, the error is frequently made with reference to the word-ending (*breakfast* for *breaking*, *jilt* for *jilted*, *because* for *beware*, *terrier* for *terror*).

Perseverations are not uncommon. Alajouanine (1968, p. 128) reports that one of his alexic patients was once requested to read aloud the following text: '*Pierre se casse une jambe. Après le jour de l'an, il fit très froid. Les enfants ne sortirent plus. La mare de la ferme gela.*' These sentences were misread as: '*Pierre se lasse dans la lance. Après le jour de l'an, la fin que les enfants ne sont plus la lance de sa lance lance sur la sur de la terre, de la terre sur ...*'

Alajouanine also remembers a patient who had the impression, when his alexia set in, that all the articles in his newspaper began with the same sentence.

Literal alexics who cannot identify a letter by sight may be able to recognize it if they are allowed to follow its contour with their finger (e.g. Péron and Goutner, 1944; Boudouresque *et al.*, 1972). This reading through kinesthesia is known as *Wilbrand's manoeuvre*. Not every pure alexic can successfully resort to kinesthetic reading, however (e.g. Ombredane, 1944).

In this connection, it should be mentioned that graphesthesia, or dermolexia, is often preserved in pure word blindness (e.g. our first case). In Lhermitte and Beauvois' patient (1973), however, it was severely disturbed.

Sometimes patients who are unable to recognize a letter can identify it if it is written in front of them, i.e. if they can see the letter being drawn. Such alexics are said to exhibit *static alexia* (e.g. Sasanuma, 1974).

It is to be noted that in literal alexia the reading of neologisms is impossible.

In pure alexia reading difficulties may vary with the system of writing. Sasanuma (1974) has reported the case of a Japanese scholar who was familiar with two orthographic systems: *kana*, which comprises symbols representing syllables, and *kanji* which is composed of symbols representing words. Following a cerebro-vascular accident, this scholar became alexic. Reading of kana words was possible only if he was allowed to apply Wilbrand's manoeuvre to the successive syllabic signs. Once the individual syllables had been kinesthetically identified, the sound pattern of the word led to the discovery of its meaning.

In kanji, the patient would either recognize the word by sight or fail to identify it altogether, for moving his finger over the strokes of the ideogram was of little avail. Thus, in kana reading was possible though it was slow and laborious. In kanji, it was rather hit or miss. Remarkably enough, compound ideograms were generally not more difficult to read than simple ones. (This was also the case with Yamadori's Japanese patient, 1975.)

Reading difficulties may also vary with the language the patient attempts to decipher. Hinshelwood (1902) has described an educated Englishman who following a cerebro-vascular accident presented a word blindness that was greatest with English – his mother-tongue – less, with French, even less with Latin, and least of all with Greek.

In a case of global alexia, Holmes (1950) noted that the patient could, in a list of four words written under one another, usually pick out the one that denoted an object presented by the examiner. Stachowiak and Poeck (1976) observed the same behaviour in a patient who was otherwise completely alexic. Replacing the object, or the picture of it, by the spoken name of the word to be picked out was even more efficient. This was also observed in the case reported by Kreindler and Ionasescu (1961).

Some alexic patients find the reading of figures as difficult as that of letters (e.g. Crouzon and Valence, 1923; Péron and Goutner, 1944). More frequently, however, the identification of digits is preserved, and the reading of numbers is generally better than that of words. Although he was severely dyslexic for written language, Ajax's first patient (1967) could deal with figures and mathematical formulas and follow a course of technical engineering.

On the other hand, the alexia may affect not only written language, including shorthand (e.g. Gloning et al., 1955), but also such graphic codes as musical notation (e.g. Dejerine, 1892). The identification of traffic signs may (e.g. our 2nd case) or may not (e.g. Warrington and Zangwill, 1957; Ajax, 1967) be disturbed. Some alexics can still read the time (e.g. Baruk et al., 1928; Warrington and Zangwill, 1957; Boucher et al., 1975); others no longer can (e.g. Fincham et al., 1975; Gloning et al., 1955).

In many cases, verbal material, although it can hardly be read, yet can easily be distinguished from non-verbal graphic symbols. Indeed, Assal and Zander's patient (1975), while he found it difficult to identify letters, yet could readily tell whether a given letter was upper- or lowercase, or whether it was presented upside down. He knew whether a given word belonged to his mother-tongue or to a foreign language, even though he could not read it. Our third case could distinguish letters which belong to the Roman alphabet from letters which do not, though he found it difficult to name any of them. The patient of Caplan and Hedley-Whyte (1974) could position individual plastic letters, without, however, being able to identify them. She could sometimes correct misspellings in words which she herself misnamed. When shown the word CATAT, she covered the last two letters, but misread the word as 'boy'. When given a list of miscellaneous words and requested to look for the name of a colour, she pointed to the word *brown* and said 'tan'. A similar behaviour has been observed in split brain patients. Commissurotomized patients may be able to identify words which are presented tachistoscopically in their left visual field, but err when they have to tell which words they have seen. They may say *clip* or *cigarette lighter* when the word that was flashed is *knife*. They have correctly read the word, though, since they can retrieve the corresponding object from a display of miscellaneous instruments. It thus appears that their right hemisphere can read isolated words but cannot name them (Sperry and Gazzaniga, 1967). Since Caplan and Hedley-Whyte's patient had a complete, congruous right hemianopia without macular sparing, she could perceive written material with her right hemisphere only. Presumably, her minor hemisphere could identify isolated words but could not name them.

Alexic patients are usually easily fatiguable, and tiredness, as was observed in Ajax's case (1967), enhances the reading difficulties and may occasionally cause perseverations in the identification of individual letters or words. Frequent rest periods increase efficiency, as was also noted by Beringer and Stein (1930).

In pure word blindness, spontaneous writing and writing under dictation are most of the time fluent and in some cases errorless. There may be omissions and iterations of words due to the inability to read over what one has written, and frequently there are reduplications of letters and of strokes (as in our first case; Michaux, Lamache et Picard, 1924; Ombredane, 1944, p. 117), due to the lack of visual control of writing (Lebrun and Lebrun, 1971). The right extremity of the lines may be slanted downwards, as in our second case.

Copying is generally laborious and faulty. In some instances, it is completely impossible (e.g. Baruk et al., 1928; Cohen et al., 1976). Occasionally, however, copying is correct (e.g. Geschwind and Fusillo, 1966; Sasanuma, 1974), although it may take more time than normal (e.g. Ajax, 1967).

As a rule, pure alexics cannot read back what they have written, once the memory of it has ceased to operate.

Benson and Geschwind (1969) are of the opinion that 'the patient with alexia without agraphia readily comprehends words spelled aloud to him by the examiner and also spells aloud correctly'. However, as our first case shows, some pure alexics do have difficulty spelling words aloud, even though they can write them properly. By contrast, there are pure alexics in whom the ability to spell aloud from memory has been remarkably preserved. Bramwell (1897) has reported a case of pure alexia, in which this ability had been so completely retained that the patient's relatives could continue to refer to her on any doubtful point of spelling.

As regards the ability to identify words spelled aloud by the examiner, it is worth mentioning that an alexic patient of Sasanuma's (1974) could recognize most kanji words that comprise several signs, when these signs and their spatial arrangement were specified to him. For instance, when told that there is an ideogram made up of the sign for *man* on the left and the sign for *book* on the right, the patient knew that this was the symbol for *body*.

Not infrequently patients with pure word blindness also exhibit some degrees of anomia (e.g. Crouzon and Valence, 1923). Sometimes they have optic aphasia, which is the inability to name objects presented visually, with preserved ability to name them as soon as they are perceived through another sensory channel, such as touch (e.g. Caplan and Hedley-Whyte, 1974). In some cases, optic aphasia is limited to images: objects can be named while their graphic representations cannot (e.g. Boudouresque *et al.*, 1972). A curious case of pure alexia with optic aphasia has been reported in detail by Lhermitte and Beauvois (1973).

In a way, pure alexia may be said to be an optic aphasia for written material; letters and/or written words can no longer be given their names. Hence the term *optic alexia* which is sometimes used as a synonym for *pure word blindness*.

Pure alexics occasionally exhibit visual agnosia: they have difficulty recognizing familiar objects perceived visually (e.g. Rubens and Benson, 1971).

Most patients with pure alexia err when they have to name colours upon confrontation or to point to colours named by the examiner. However, the majority of them match colours correctly and can adequately answer such questions as *What is the colour of snow?* or *What is the colour of blood?* What they fail to do properly is, in fact, to match colours with their verbal labels. These patients thus have what Geschwind and Fusillo (1966) have called *colour-name aphasia*, but they do not have colour agnosia. Unfortunately, this distinction is not always made in neurological papers.

It is noteworthy that in Ombredane's case (1944) there was some degree of colour agnosia (which was apparent when the patient had to classify shades of a colour) but no colour-name aphasia.

In pure alexics verbal short-term memory may be reduced, as in our third case, who could not recall brief stories. Crouzon and Valence (1923) noted that their patient could not remember verbal instructions.

Some pure alexics (e.g. Caplan and Hedley-Whyte, 1974) are reported to have finger agnosia. It is not always clear, however, what impairment these patients actually exhibit, for in neurological literature the term *finger agnosia* is often used ambiguously. It may mean that the patient cannot adequately use tactile and proprioceptive information to differentiate between his fingers or to appreciate their relative position when vision is excluded; or it may mean that the patient cannot properly name fingers or indicate fingers named by the examiner. Gerstmann, who introduced the term *finger agnosia* in 1924, used it initially to denote the inability to deal appropriately with the names of the fingers. Later he extended his conception considerably and by 1957 he was using *finger agnosia* to refer to the inability to recognize, identify, differentiate, name, select or indicate the individual fingers of either hand. As a matter of fact, only the loss of the ability to identify the individual fingers independently of language should be called *finger agnosia*. The impairment to which Gerstmann originally applied the term *finger agnosia* is verbal in nature and should be called *finger aphasia*. It is essential to carefully distinguish between the two disorders, as patients with true finger agnosia generally have no finger aphasia, while many aphasics have difficulty naming fingers or indicating fingers named but do not evidence finger agnosia (Kinsbourne and Warrington, 1962). Whether a number of pure alexics have true finger agnosia or an isolated finger aphasia is an unsettled matter, due to the confused terminology.

In a number of cases (e.g. Levine and Calvanio, 1978), simultanagnosia accompanies alexia. Because he was so engrossed in punctual details, Ombredane's patient (1944, pp. 90–91) found it easier to identify normally drawn figures than figures made up of discrete points (as in Ishiara's test). Simultanagnosia may be the reason why some alexics identify isolated letters more readily than groups of letters, i.e. words.

In some pure alexics, calculating ability is preserved (e.g. Dejerine, 1892; Crouzon and Valence, 1923); in others it is impaired (as in our first two cases or in Warrington and Zangwill, 1957).

A disorder of topographical orientation is often found. Our first two cases showed this handicap. Ombredane's patient (1944, pp. 100–101) also.

Martin (1954) considered pure word blindness to result from a disturbance of visual space perception. Accordingly, he held that pure alexics have difficulty identifying geometric forms. However, as Péron and Goutner's case (1944) demonstrates, recognition of geometric shapes may be totally preserved. Immediate recall of geometric designs proved unabated in the patient described by Ajax *et al.* (1977).

On the other hand, drawing may be impaired, as in Kreindler and Ionasescu's case (1961).

Patients with pure word alexia generally have right homonymous hemianopia, but a few cases have been reported (e.g. Péron and Goutner, 1944; Greenblatt, 1973) in which no visual field defect could be detected. In Ombredane's case (1944, p. 88), the ophthalmologist reported no hemianopia, but the patient complained that vision tended to be blurred in the right visual field.

On the other hand, motor or somatosensory disorders are generally mild, if present at all.

It appears from the foregoing that patients with pure alexia do not by any means present a uniform syndrome. The severity of the reading disturbance, the kind of material that can no longer be deciphered, the facilitating circumstances, and the concomitant disorders may vary considerably from patient to patient.

Despite its variability, the syndrome of pure alexia nearly always results from a lesion affecting the splenium of the corpus callosum and parts of the occipital lobe in the dominant hemisphere. Most of the time this lesion destroys the left visual cortex or the optic radiations to it, and severs the right visual cortex from the left angular gyrus, which is pivotal in the decoding of written language. Sometimes, the left calcarine fissure and the optic radiations to it are spared, but the pathways from both visual cortices to the left angular gyrus are cut off. In either case, pure alexia may be considered a disconnection syndrome, as was suggested by Dejerine as early as 1892 and later emphasized by Geschwind (1962). A few cases have been reported, however, in which the left occipital lobe and the fibers leading from it to the angular gyrus had been preserved (e.g. Fincham *et al.*, 1975). In such cases, the pathophysiology of pure alexia is difficult to explain.

On the other hand, recent anatomo-clinical reports by Ajax *et al.* (1977) and by Vincent *et al.* (1977) suggest that when pure alexia is not accompanied by colour-name aphasia the dorsal or superior fibres of the splenium are likely to have been spared.

3

DELAYED AUDITORY FEEDBACK: A POSSIBLE CLUE TO THE MECHANISM OF SOME TYPES OF APHASIA

FRANÇOIS BOLLER

Delayed Auditory Feedback (DAF) is widely known for its disruptive effect on the speech of normal subjects. Normals in most cases react to DAF by speaking more loudly and slowly and by showing qualitative changes in verbal output.

Little research, however, has been done on the effect of DAF in patients with localized hemispheric damage and particularly in those with aphasia. In this paper I wish to discuss some recent investigations performed with my collaborators at the Neurobehavior Unit of the Cleveland VA Hospital, Drs. P. Bart Vrtunski, James L. Mack and Youngjai Kim. We have been studying DAF in patients with aphasia. We consider DAF to be an experimental tool, with the property of modifying both speech and language. We believe that our experiments may lead to a better understanding of both aphasia and language.

It was as early as 1932 that Kern, a speech pathologist, stressed the need to examine the feedback actions occurring as a result of the auditory perception of speech, and the possible relationship between auditory stimulation and stammering. Kern found that stammering decreased markedly or stopped altogether when stammerers read a passage while a white noise was fed into their ears. Then, in 1950 and 1951, respectively, Lee and Black offered the first formal descriptions of the DAF effect. Since those early studies, a good deal of additional work reporting various effects of DAF in normals and stutterers has been performed (see Yates, 1963 for a review).

In 1955 Birch and Lee used a technique similar to the one Kern used in 1932: a white noise was fed into the ears of patients with expressive aphasia. Birch and Lee claimed that this 'noisy environment' improved the performance of aphasics, although their findings were later strongly contradicted by Weinstein (1959).

Stanton, a neurologist from Edinburgh, was probably the first to systematically study the effect of DAF in aphasics (1958). He asked 13 aphasic patients to read a text and recite a nursery rhyme. Although we are not given many details about the extent and severity of their aphasia, 'routine tests for aphasia' found most of them to be 'suffering from either a predominantly expressive aphasia or a mixed expressive and receptive aphasia', according to the nomenclature of Weisenburg and MacBride (1935). Stanton adopted a system of scoring in which disturbances 'known to be caused by DAF in normal subjects' were each scored on a three-point scale of intensity. These disturbances included alterations of stress, disturbance of rhythm, lengthening of vowel sound duration, reduplication of consonants, syllables, and words, and substitution of wrong consonants, syllables, and words. Changes in vocal intensity, in pitch, and in voice intonation were not taken into account. Performance without DAF was compared to subsequent performance with DAF. Stanton found that the 13 patients tested fell into four main groups: (1) those who responded to DAF in a manner similar to that of normal subjects (3 patients); (2) those who appeared to be unaffected by DAF (2 patients); (3) those in whom speech appeared to be improved in some ways under DAF conditions (5 patients); and (4) a fourth group of patients whose response to DAF was atypical: in two of these three patients, the effect of DAF appeared to be to 'lock' the speech utterance to a low but marked rhythm, within which each vowel sound was intensely prolonged and uttered on a rising note.

The three patients who had a 'normal' effect had predominantly expressive speech disturbances and showed the least evidence of any receptive disorder. Stanton postulated that such patients retain a functioning auditory monitoring system susceptible to disturbance by DAF, and he concluded that the basis of their speech disorder 'lies in a disturbance of some other part of the speech mechanism' (perhaps the kinesthetic monitoring system). Patients who were unaffected by DAF were thought to have a defective or absent auditory monitoring mechanism. Such patients may suffer a concomitant disturbance of both kinesthetic and auditory feedback. Stanton's patients had mixed or receptive aphasia and were tested

96

soon (less than a week) after stroke. As for the patients who appeared to be improved by DAF, Stanton suspected that the experimental technique perhaps reinforced 'an attenuated normal feedback activity which is not strong enough alone to monitor speech effectively.' On the other hand, this phenomenon could be the result of 'abolishing inhibitory influences arising in the auditory centers' as Birch and Lee (1955) suggested when explaining the effect they had found. Stanton apparently found no patient with a DAF effect greater than normal. His paper, however, was the first to mention the possibility that some aphasics have a DAF effect strikingly different from that in normals and other aphasics.

In 1964, Alajouanine, Lhermitte, Ledoux, Renaud, and Vignolo studied two groups of patients with jargon aphasia. In the first group, the paraphasias consisted almost exclusively of phonemic substitutions ('phonemic jargon'); the second group showed almost exclusively word substitutions ('verbal jargon'). Neither group showed dysarthria, buccofacial apraxia, auditory agnosia, or a severe impairment of comprehension. Both groups were given a battery of tests which included DAF. The speech production tasks consisted of counting from 1 to 30 and reciting the alphabet, the days of the week, the months, and a prayer or a piece of poetry they knew by heart. Finally, reading aloud and spontaneous speech were compared. The score was based on surprise reactions, blocking, repetitions and skipping, and a slowdown in speech rate. As in Stanton's study, changes in intensity were not taken into account. None of Alajouanine's 19 patients with phonemic jargon showed language changes under DAF. They could count and recite without rate changes and without blocking repetitions or skipping phonemes. There wasn't even a surprise reaction. However, patients with semantic paraphasias were all as disturbed as normal subjects.

Alajouanine *et al.* (1964) interpreted these and other of their findings as supportive of their hypothesis that two separate systems are implicated in comprehension. The first is a sensorimotor, auditory-phonemic system responsible for the production and reception of phonemic units. An impairment in this system not only produces phonemic jargon but also affects auditory perception at the phonemic level, with impairment of phonemic discrimination, loss of the DAF effect, and deficits in the translation of auditory sequences into manual ones. The second system, the semantic one, is thought to control the process of connecting thought and language, and a disturbance in this system results in the production of semantic jargon and the impairment of semantic comprehension.

In 1969 Singh and Schlanger studied the effect of DAF in 3 groups of handicapped subjects: 10 aphasics, 10 dysarthrics, and 10 mentally retarded. Duration (i.e., time needed to read sentences) differed significantly in the three groups. Two aphasic subjects had a shorter duration under DAF: one of these was 'expressive–receptive' and the other was a 'severe expressive'. Another aphasic patient was unaffected by DAF. Singh and Schlanger noticed that 'the deleterious effect of delayed sidetone was significantly less on the aphasic subjects than on the dysarthric or mentally retarded subjects.' These data would be easier to interpret had more details been given about the type of aphasia of Singh's subjects and had a normal control group been included. One additional study should be mentioned here; in 1974, Heilman reported that some patients with severe Wernicke's aphasia showed no detectable changes in their spontaneous output under DAF.

The fact that the foregoing brief review covers much of the available literature on the effect of DAF in aphasics gives some indication of why we felt the need for a systematic study of DAF effects in patients with hemispheric lesions. The present paper is based on material published elsewhere (Vrtunski, Mack, Boller, and Kim, 1976; Boller, Vrtunski, Kim, and Mack, 1978) and on work currently in progress in our laboratory (Kim, Bonstelle, Royer and Boller, 1979; Vrtunski, Martinez, and Boller, in press).

In a preliminary study (Vrtunski et al., 1976), we used an objective method of recording and measuring intensity and duration induced by DAF in patients with unilateral hemispheric damage. Figure 1 shows the increase induced by DAF in both intensity and duration. Our study indicated that all subjects (including those with aphasia) showed a DAF effect. However, the DAF effect in aphasics appeared to be different from that in normals and in right-hemisphere-damaged patients.

A subsequent study (Boller et al., 1978) focused in greater detail on DAF and aphasia. On the basis of a short aphasia battery, we subdivided aphasic patients into 2 groups, 10 with non-fluent (Broca's) and 10 with fluent aphasia, and compared their performance to that of 10 normal controls. The patients with fluent aphasia were further

98

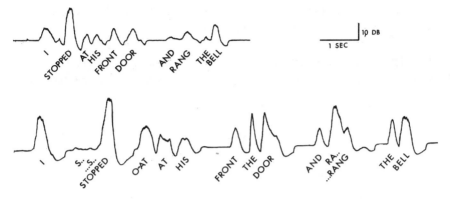

Figure 1. Strip chart recording of a right-hemisphere-damaged subject reading a sentence. The upper tracing is without DAF, the lower tracing is under DAF conditions. (From Vrtunski *et al.*, *Cortex*, *12*: 395–404, 1976, by permission.)

subdivided (Figure 2) into one of four subtypes: (1) Wernicke's aphasia (fluent aphasia with poor repetition and comprehension, 4 patients); (2) Conduction aphasia (fluent aphasia with good comprehension and a severe repetition disturbance, 3 patients); (3) Word deafness (poor auditory comprehension and relatively preserved reading comprehension, 2 patients); and (4) Transcortical sensory aphasia (fluent aphasia with good repetition but a marked impairment in comprehension, 1 patient).

Each subject was given six speech production tasks: (1) repeating sounds and words; (2) naming objects; (3) producing sentences from given stimulus words; (4) answering questions; (5) reciting nursery rhymes; and (6) reading. Two delays were used, 180 and 360 msec. Two independent judges rated patients' responses in terms of three variables: intensity, duration, and the quality of speech. For each variable, the judges were asked to state whether the performance under DAF was the same or different from that without DAF (referred to as Simultaneous Auditory Feedback, SAF). For quality of speech, a score of -1 reflected an improvement in the way the patient spoke; a score of 1 was given for a phonemic substitution or any other minor change in the quality of the utterance; a score of 2 was given when the word or utterance was severely distorted but still recognizable; and a score of 3 was given when the word or utterance could not be recognized or a different word was used. Inter-judge reliability was considered sufficiently high to justify the pooling of two judges' ratings into one score. Rating for intensity and duration followed an approximately similar criterion.

Results can be summarized as follows: all subjects showed at least some DAF effect (Figure 2). As Figure 3 shows, the three groups

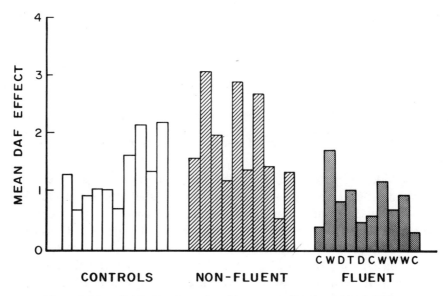

Figure 2. Mean DAF effect for each subject across all tasks and both delays. Drawn from data of Boller *et al.*, 1978.

differed significantly; as a group, the non-fluent aphasics tended to show a significantly greater DAF effect than did the fluent aphasics, and the normal controls fell somewhere in between. The three indices of DAF (intensity, duration, and quality of speech, shown as separate segments in the columns of Figure 3) differ in their ability to discriminate among the three groups. While changes in intensity were not statistically different among the groups, quality of speech definitely differentiated in all three, with the non-fluent aphasics showing a greater effect than normals and fluent aphasics showing a significantly smaller DAF effect than normals with this criterion. Changes in duration were also greater in non-fluent than in fluent aphasics.

In general, as Figure 3 shows, the 180 msec delay produced a greater DAF effect than did the 360 msec interval.

There was considerable variability in the DAF effect induced by

100

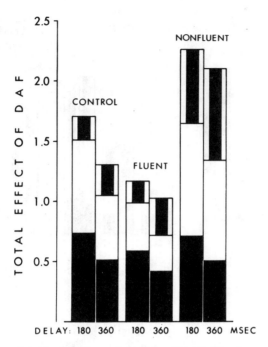

Figure 3: Overall DAF effect for each group and DAF delay in msec. Each column consists of three parts, corresponding to 'Intensity' (bottom, black), 'Duration' (middle, white), and 'Quality of Speech' (top, black and white) changes. There is a highly significant difference between the two aphasic groups for both delay intervals. (Reprinted from Boller *et al.*, 1978, by permission.)

each task, as can be seen in Figure 4A and B. An interesting result can be seen in reading, where the fluent aphasics under DAF read more loudly and slowly, but the quality of their reading actually improved (as shown by the 'quality' measure situated below the zero line in Figure 4). We found, in addition, that repeating a polysyllabic word ('frustration') elicited a significantly greater DAF effect than repeating a simple sound ('ah'). In other tasks, however, this 'subtask effect' was not apparent. For example, reading a tongue twister did not produce a significantly greater DAF effect than did reading 'Mary had a little lamb'.

The fact that all patients included in this study showed at least some DAF effect confirms the results of one previous study (Vrtunski *et al.*, 1976) but contrasts with the findings of other investigators (e.g., Stanton, 1958 and Heilman, 1974) who noted that some aphasics failed to show any detectable DAF effect. This difference in results is

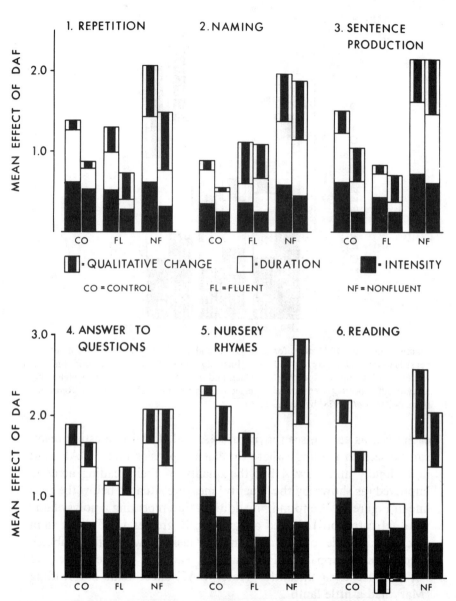

Figure 4. DAF effect for each group, DAF delay, and task. (CO=Controls; FL=Fluent aphasics; NF=Non-fluent aphasics. (Reprinted from Boller *et al.*, 1978, by permission.)

probably not due to a difference in patients in the studies (our patients presented a wide range in both type and severity of aphasia), but rather to the fact that we used more rigorous and better-specified criteria for judging the presence of DAF.

We did find that different types of aphasics vary widely in the amount of changes induced by DAF. Patients with non-fluent (Broca's) aphasia showed the greatest DAF effect. Although we do not have sufficient data to clearly explain this result, it could be due to a non-specific effect of DAF: patients who are already struggling to talk might be hampered by any distracting stimulus. However, other investigators have found that language is not impaired by a white noise, and it has even been claimed that under such conditions, the language of expressive aphasics tends to improve (Birch and Lee, 1955). We thus hypothesize, rather, that this result is a specific effect of DAF and suggest that perhaps Broca's aphasics rely more heavily on auditory feedback than do normal subjects. It would be interesting to measure the correlation between DAF and recovery from aphasia. Stanton (1958) states that his two patients who were unaffected by DAF were tested soon after the onset of aphasia. It is possible that among non-fluent aphasics, an improvement in aphasia might be accompanied by a gradually increasing DAF effect. This hypothesis could not be tested in our sample since all our patients had had aphasia for some time. If, in the course of further study, we were able to confirm this hypothesis, DAF could be used as an easily quantifiable measurement of recovery from Broca's aphasia.

The finding that fluent aphasics show a smaller DAF effect than do normals is compatible with the idea that fluent aphasics suffer from a defect in feedback. Disturbance in auditory feedback has long been suspected as the cause of the discrepancy in fluent aphasics between the apparent lack of concern for their own often incomprehensible output and the surprise they show when they hear their own previously tape-recorded output (Alajouanine, Sabouraud and de Ribaucourt, 1952) or other meaningless utterances (Boller and Green, 1972).

Figure 2 shows that three patients with conduction aphasia in our study were responsible in large part for the differences between the fluent group and the normal controls.

In fact, the conduction aphasics showed a significantly smaller DAF effect than did the four patients with Wernicke's aphasia (p<.05 by the Wilcoxon Rank Sum Test). Comparison of the 3 conduction aphasics and the other 7 patients included in the 'fluent' group showed an even greater difference (p<.01). Conversely, when the three conduction aphasics were removed from the fluent group and the seven remaining patients were compared with the normal controls, the difference between the two groups was no longer significant (p=.10).

The group that Alajouanine et al. (1964) found to have no DAF effect (fluent aphasics with phonemic jargon) shows several characteristics of what we call conduction aphasia. Our results, therefore, are compatible with those investigators' hypothesis that these patients have a specific phonemic impairment, not only in their output but in auditory input as well.

As can be seen in Figure 2, one patient with Broca's aphasia in our study showed very little DAF effect, while one patient with Wernicke's aphasia had a considerable DAF effect. Review of these patients' records showed that the diagnosis, as far as the type of aphasia was concerned, was undoubtedly correct. Both patients had had a CT scan and, as can be seen, the patient with Broca's aphasia and little DAF effect had a left temporal lobe lesion (Figure 5). The patient with Wernicke's aphasia had a lesion in the left Wernicke's area, but his lesion appeared to extend into the frontal lobe (Figure 6A and B). Of all the other patients, only one, a patient with word deafness and bilateral temporal lobe lesion, had had a CT scan. It is therefore impossible to speculate on the significance of the above data, except to say that perhaps what matters is not so much the type of aphasia but the anatomical site of the lesion. Studies currently in progress (Naeser, Hayward and Zatz, 1976; Kim et al., 1979) will help to clarify the relationship between anatomical locus of lesion and the type of neuropsychological symptoms encountered in each patient.

A final point should be made regarding the criteria used to measure the amount of changes induced by DAF. In our first study (Vrtunski et al., 1976), these changes were recorded and measured objectively; most of the results discussed in this paper, however, were based on the subjective ratings of two independent judges. We (Vrtunski, Martinez and Boller, in press) are now in the process of comparing an objective method of estimating one of the parameters of the DAF effect (duration) with the subjective rating given by two judges on the same parameter. We have calculated the coefficient of correlation between the objective and the subjective methods of rating. For the 180 msec delay, the interval often found to produce

104

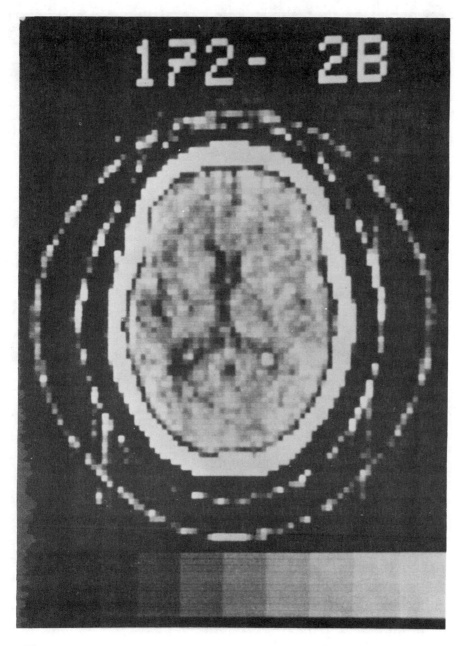

Figure 5. CT scan of a patient with Broca's aphasia and a small DAF effect. Lesion is in the anterior part of the left temporal lobe (EMI scan done at the Cleveland Clinic).

105

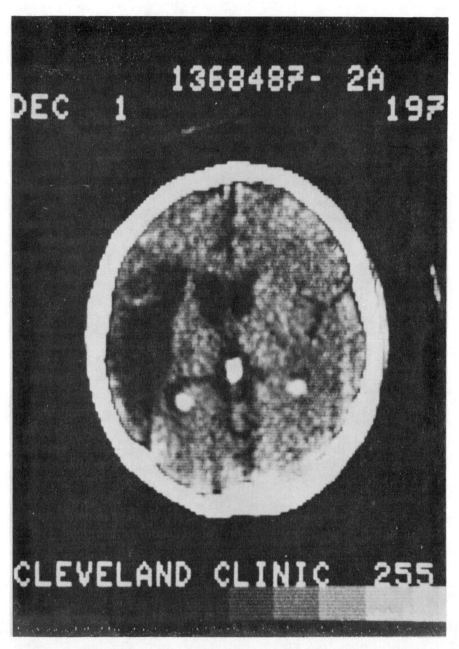

Figure 6A. CT scan of a patient with Wernicke's aphasia and a large DAF effect. The lesion extends to the left frontal lobe (EMI scan done at the Cleveland Clinic).

106

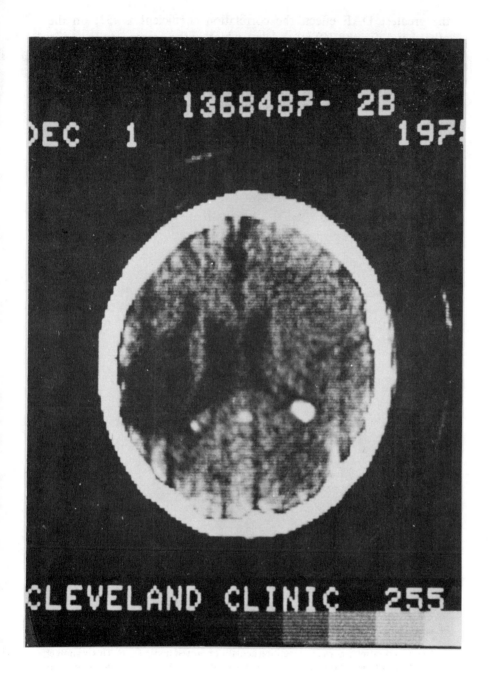

Figure 6B.

the greatest DAF effect, the correlation coefficient is .52; on the other hand, for the 360 msec delay, which in the present study and in several previous ones was found to produce a less clear-cut DAF effect, the correlation coefficient between the objective and the subjective rating is .46. These values, although not very high, are statistically significant. Further work is currently in progress to elucidate the significance of these results.*

* After submission of this manuscript, Boller and Marcie (1978) described a patient with conduction aphasia whose repetition actually improved under DAF. This is another data in favor of the hypothesis that abnormal auditory feedback may play a role in the pathogenesis of conduction aphasia.

4

VERBAL EXPRESSION AND EXPRESSIVE PANTOMIME IN APHASIC PATIENTS

SUE ANDERSON DAVIS, RICHARD ARTES,
RICHARD HOOPS

Literature regarding aphasia indicates considerable disagreement as to how gesture and pantomime are affected by higher cortical damage. As early as 1819, Combe published a collection of essays on phrenology citing a man who 'spoke incoherently and forgot names of words, yet gesture was eloquently retained' (Critchley, 1970).

In 1870, Finkelnburg described 'asymbolia' as a 'generalized disturbance in the capacity to express or comprehend symbols through any modality, including gesture and pantomime' (Bay, 1964).

Pick (1931) proposed that gesture and pantomime were commonly exaggerated in cases of severe aphemia as a compensation for impaired verbal expressive abilities. He asserted that receptive comprehension could be aided through the use of the gestural modality. Critchley (1939) reported that the aphasic patient can usually express himself clearly by pantomime after suffering a gross reduction in available vocabulary. He further stated that the pantomime may lack its normal richness and complexity as a consequence of the cerebral accident, yet meanings of the pantomimic communications are retained despite possible involvements of the upper extremity. Critchley found that in the vast majority of aphasics, verbal speech suffered considerably more than gestural language.

Goldstein (1948) concurred with Critchley and further observed that patients suffering from different forms of aphasia varied as to the appearance of their gestures. In some cases of aphasia, gestures and pantomime were highly exaggerated. Brain (1961) also saw a tendency for gestural communication to be superior to that of verbal utterances, particularly in cases of jargon and nominal aphasia. Cases of highly expressive pantomime in jargon aphasia were documented by Alajouanine and Lhermitte (1964) as they noted a significance in the nonverbal communication which had been missing in oral speech. Patients with motor or Broca's aphasia were found to utilize very poor gestures; however, temporal aphasics demonstrated rich and increasingly complex gesticulation.

The effect of aphasia on the sign language of deaf individuals was investigated in two separate studies within recent literature. Osgood and Miron (1963) found that sign language of deaf mutes with left cerebral lesions was highly vulnerable to aphasia. A case study conducted by Sarno, Swisher, and Sarno (1969) documented the control of communication processes in the dominant hemisphere. The deaf patient's recovery of his rudimentary speech utterances and basic signs prior to his fingerspelling ability provided support for the theory of recovering effective speech prior to the other language processes.

The first evaluative instrument to include assessment of pantomimic abilities of aphasic patients was developed by Eisenson (1954). Although only minimal gestural skills were tested, the task required the aphasic to pantomime certain routine daily activities. Porch (1967) developed a more comprehensive battery for evaluation of the aphasic which included gestural tasks along with verbal and graphic skills. Gesture and the use of pantomime were evaluated through eight separate tasks covering various levels of difficulty.

As indicated, a number of authorities have observed that aphasics demonstrate impaired nonverbal behaviors, yet only three extensive experimental studies have investigated the degree of gestural and pantomimic impairment in aphasics.

Goodglass and Kaplan (1963) administered an extensive test of gesture and pantomime to a group of 20 aphasic patients and a group of 19 non-aphasic brain-injured patients who were closely matched in both age and intellectual efficiency. Forty-six different items were utilized within the testing of five types of gestural movement ranging from the description of objects to the performance of related sequences of events. In each task, the examiner gave the subject verbal instructions to perform certain gestural sequences. Responses were scored on three levels of adequacy in addition to a number of qualitative categories including gestural enhancement, pantomimed context, verbal overflow, and body-part as object. The authors reported the following conclusions:

(1) Aphasics have a gestural deficiency which is best understood as an apractic disorder consequent to left hemisphere lesion; the concept of a general communication disorder is not supported. The bases for this conclusion are:

(a) Aphasics were inferior in gestural ability to their intellectual counterparts in a control group at each level of intellectual efficiency.

(b) Aphasics were less able to profit from the opportunity to imitate than were the non-aphasic controls.

(c) When the influence of auditory comprehension was controlled, gestural ability was not related to the severity of aphasia.

(d) In the absence of aphasia, left hemisphere lesions produced more impaired movements than did the right hemisphere lesions.

(2) Gestural ability is impaired in direct relation to the loss of intellectual efficiency in brain-injured patients, whether aphasic or otherwise.

Pickett (1972) investigated the relationship between gesture and aphasia through the development of an experimental test battery. Eight tasks were designed to test tactile recognition, pantomimic expression, gestural recognition, and imitative ability of aphasic patients. Tasks utilized ten objects with predominantly verbal instructions. After standardization of materials and procedures on a normal population, the experimental test battery and the Porch Index of Communicative Ability (PICA) were administered to 28 aphasic patients. Responses were scored according to the PICA system of multidimensional choices. Following use of these procedures, Pickett concluded that:

(1) The experimental test was a successful and reliable instrument for measuring the gestural ability of aphasic patients.

(2) Gestural ability was related to the overall severity of aphasia.

(3) The explanation of gestural deficit resulting from limb apraxia is not supported.

Duffy, Duffy and Pearson (1975) looked at the extent of the impairment of pantomime recognition in addition to the relationship between pantomime recognition and verbal deficits in aphasia. Subjects were divided into four groups consisting of aphasics, right-hemisphere damaged, subcortically damaged, and normals. Each subject was administered the Pantomime Recognition Test and three tests of verbal ability including the Naming Test, the Verbal Recognition Test, and the PICA. The Pantomime recognition was established by having the patient point to the appropriate picture as the examiner pantomimed the use of a particular object. Verbal ability was then evaluated through both receptive recognition and expressive naming. The PICA was used as a general measure of language impairment. Results of the study indicated a greater impairment in pantomime recognition of the aphasics than in the other groups of subjects. High correlations were also found between the impairment of pantomime recognition and the impaired verbal ability in aphasics. Aphasia was thus supported as a general impairment of symbolic communication presenting nonverbal as well as verbal deficits.

Procedure
Twenty normal subjects and twenty aphasic subjects participated in this study. Normal subjects with no history or medical evidence of neurological damage were chosen from a random population. The thirteen males and seven females were then divided into two groups according to age. The ten subjects in normal group A ranged in age from 20 to 49 years with a mean age of 29.4 years, while the ten subjects in normal group B ranged in age from 50 to 80 years with a .nean age of 64.0 years. The overall mean age of the normal subjects was 46.7 years. The mean level of education was 12.4 years.

Aphasic subjects were chosen from four convalescent centres located in the same geographical area of northeastern and east central Indiana. Subjects who had medical evidence of left hemisphere cerebral vascular accident (CVA) as indicated on current medical records by the attending physician and who demonstrated aphasic symptoms as determined by the resident speech pathologist were classified as 'aphasics' for the purposes of this study. Subjects were excluded on the basis of a history of psychiatric problems, bilateral limb involvement which would interfere with gestural capacity, visual acuity problems (with the exception of right homonymous hemianopsia), hearing acuity problems which interfered with the reception of verbal directions, or complete inability to perform on either the verbal or the pantomime portions of the test.

Experimental subjects ranged in age from 58 to 83 years with a mean age of 73.3 years. Although prior studies in the area have suggested a higher prevalence of aphasia in males than in females

(Schuell, 1964; Eisenson, 1973), the aphasic population in the four convalescent centres selected for this study yielded 3 males and 17 females as subjects. Right hemiplegia was evident in 16 subjects with no hemiplegia in 4 subjects. Months post onset of the cerebral vascular accident ranged from 4 to 105 months with a mean of 29.7 months. Subjects had a mean level of education of 12.1 years.

Table 1. *Data descriptive of the age, education, and sex of aphasic and normal subjects; and data descriptive of months post onset and incidence of right hemiplegia in aphasic subjects*

Subjects	Age in Years			Years Education			Sex	
	Mean	SD	Range	Mean	SD	Range	Male	Female
Aphasic N=20	73.3	6.7	58–83	12.1	3.0	8–16	7	13
Normal N=20	46.7	20.6	20–80	12.4	2.8	8–16	3	17
Group A N=10	29.4	9.4	20–49					
Group B N=10	64.0	11.9	50–80					

	Months Post Onset			Hemiplegic	
	Mean	SD	Range	Yes	No
Aphasic N=20	29.7	22.8	4–105	16	4

In selecting the subjects for this investigation, no attempt was made to restrict the degree of severity nor to eliminate subjects who demonstrated the presence of mild dysarthrias or apraxias. If such problems prevented performance of either verbal or pantomimic tasks, testing was terminated under the guideline stated previously of complete inability to perform; however, the presence of such factors to a degree which only impaired skills in one or both modalities was considered to typify a more realistic aphasic syndrome which frequently presents such complications.

Testing was performed in rooms free of noise and distraction. All subjects were seated with a table placed before them for the presentation of stimuli. Prior to testing, each individual was engaged in a conversation as the purpose of the test was explained. At this time, a gross assessment was made of hearing, vision, and peripheral sensory acuity.

Test items consisted of fourteen colored drawings picturing common objects which had uses that could be expressed both verbally and pantomimically. Drawings of a hammer and nail, a knife and fork, a folded newspaper, and a lock and key were used to acquaint subjects with the required task. Stimulus items for the verbal and pantomime tests included: a paring knife and apple; a coffeepot and cup; a suitcase; a telephone; a pen and paper; a belt; a comb; a toothbrush and toothpaste; a letter, envelope, and stamp; and a camera. The use of homogeneous test items has proven to be advantageous in making cross-modality comparisons as well as eliminating any variation between subtests due to unfamiliar or difficult stimuli (Porch, 1967; Pickett, 1972).

The series of pictures was shown to each subject under two conditions. In Condition One, the subject received the instruction, 'As completely as possible, *tell* me what you do with (*name of object*)' as the picture was presented. Additional cues of 'what do you do with it', 'how do you use that', and '*tell* me', were given no more than twice if the subject requested a repetition, made no response within 30 seconds, or indicated that he had not understood the directions by responding inappropriately. Condition Two utilized presentation of the same pictures with the instructions, 'As completely as possible, *show* me what you do with (*name of object*)'. Additional cues of 'pretend you're using that', 'what do you do with it', and '*show* me', were given no more than twice if the subject requested a repetition, gave no response after 30 seconds, or indicated that he did not understand the directions by responding inappropriately. Pantomime accompanied the verbal instructions for each task in accordance with the finding of Fordyce and Jones (1966) that right hemiplegic patients score significantly higher when instructed by pantomime than when instructed orally for the same tasks. Conditions One and Two were administered in counterbalanced order with random presentation of stimulus items to avoid possible ordering effects.

The first four stimuli within each condition served as pretest training items to insure that each subject comprehended the task prior to administration of actual test items. Following instructions for the first pretest item, the examiner performed the initial task and asked the subject to imitate his example. Instructions were then given for pretest items two, three, and four as the subject was provided adequate time to respond. If no response was attempted within 30 seconds, if the subject requested a repetition of instructions, or if he indicated that he did not understand the task, the directions were repeated. If an inaccurate response was still produced, open-ended sentences were given to provide the subject with cues. If cues were required on all four pretest items, each item was then presented a second time without cueing. Failure to respond spontaneously to at least two of the four pretest items resulted in exclusion from the test population. Patients who performed adequately on pretest items proceeded with the test itself receiving periodic praise for effort and cooperation on all test items.

Responses were scored using the multidimensional binary choice system of the PICA (Porch, 1967) following a design which describes each response in several dimensions by assigning a single score. According to Porch (1971), 'The aphasiology literature over the past 50 years has given clear evidence that the aphasic patient's response must be described multidimensionally.' Although several methods have been developed to describe aphasic responses, the PICA system provides the greatest amount of information by specifying the nature and severity of the communication deficit while maintaining a level of complexity that is workable and efficient (Porch, 1971; Davis and Leach, 1972; Pickett, 1972).

As subjects identified the functions of stimulus items verbally and pantomimically, responses were transcribed as given. Numerical rankings on a 16-point scale were then assigned to the specific responses based on the five dimensions of accuracy, responsiveness, completeness, promptness, and efficiency. The transcriptions of each subject's responses were again scored two days later to assure reliable scoring of precise responses.

Item analyses and frequency scores were statistically determined for both the verbal expression and the expressive pantomime versions of the procedure using Crombach's Alpha to establish internal consistency and reliability for the evaluative instrument. According to Smith (1970), 'A test which is used to differentiate between individuals should have a reliability of .90 or better; but, if a test is merely intended to differentiate between the means of two or more groups, a reliability in the neighborhood of .80 is adequate.' Although the reliability coefficient for the verbal scale (0.94747) proved to be better than that for the pantomime scale (0.83858), both subtests demonstrated internal consistency and reliability.

The null hypothesis was that no differences would exist between verbal expression and expressive pantomime in either normal or aphasic subjects. In order to establish the fact that performance levels were based upon the presence of aphasia rather than concurrent factors of age or months post onset of stroke, accumulated data was interpreted with a univariate and multivariate analysis of variance, covariance, and regression using planned comparisons for the variables of age and months post onset within the groups of normal and aphasic subjects respectively. Differences in performance levels were then determined using a .05 level of significance for rejection of the null hypothesis.

Results

Presented in Table 2 are the scores from both the Verbal Expression and the Expressive Pantomime subtests for the normal and aphasic subjects. With 160 possible points on each subtest, both groups of

Table 2. *Mean test scores for normal and aphasic subjects*

Subjects		Verbal Expression	Expressive Pantomime	Total Score	Difference in Scores
Normal Subjects N=20	Mean	144.3	145.5	290.5	1.1
	SD	12.9	9.7	17.2	10.2
	Range	102–159	125–157	237–316	1–20
Aphasic Subjects N=20	Mean	93.4	132.4	225.6	35.0
	SD	22.0	14.6	32.3	20.1
	Range	62–129	91–155	174–284	8–78

subjects achieved higher scores on the pantomimic tasks than on the verbal tasks; however, the scores of the normal subjects exceeded those of the aphasic subjects in verbal expression (mean of normal subjects=144.3, mean of aphasic subjects=93.4) as well as in expressive pantomime (mean of normal subjects=145.5, mean of aphasic subjects=132.4). Mean scores from both subtests were then computed for each group to arrive at a total score as well as determining the difference between scores achieved on the Verbal Expression subtest and the Expressive Pantomime subtest. In addition to the lower total score for aphasic subjects (total score=225.6) as compared to normal subjects (total score=290.5), the difference between the two subtest scores was considerably larger for the aphasic patients (difference between scores=35.0) than for normal subjects (difference between scores=1.1). Means are also provided in Tables 3 and 4 to illustrate

116

Table 3. *Mean test scores for normal subgroups by age*

Subjects		Verbal Expression	Expressive Pantomime	Total Score	Difference in Scores
Age 20 to 49 years N=10	Mean	148.4	149.1	297.5	0.7
	SD	6.8	5.5	10.7	6.2
	Range	141–157	142–156	283–313	1–20
Age 50 to 80 years N=10	Mean	140.9	142.5	283.5	1.6
	SD	15.9	11.5	23.8	14.4
	Range	102–159	125–157	237–316	1–13

Table 4. *Mean test scores for aphasic subgroups by months post onset*

Subjects		Verbal Expression	Expressive Pantomime	Total Score	Difference in Scores
MPO less than 12 N=5	Mean	86.0	128.6	214.6	42.6
	SD	24.3	23.7	39.9	26.6
	Range	69–128	91–153	174–281	8–75
MPO 12 through 24 N=6	Mean	105.5	133.0	238.5	27.5
	SD	19.1	12.9	29.6	13.7
	Range	85–129	119–155	207–184	9–51
MPO more than 24 N=9	Mean	89.4	134.1	223.6	44.7
	SD	21.6	10.7	27.5	20.1
	Range	62–120	117–151	181–239	18–78

the individual subtest scores, total scores, and differences between the subtest scores for the normal and aphasic groups according to age and months post onset respectively.

Table 5 illustrates the planned comparisons of the summed scores and the differences between scores through analysis of variance for normal subjects according to age, for aphasic subjects by months post onset of stroke, and for the aphasic patients as compared to the normal subjects. There was no significant difference (.05 level of significance) between the performances of normal subjects from age 20 to 49 years and those from age 50 to 80 years. Aphasic subjects varying in months post onset from less than 12 months, between 12 and 24 months, and more than 24 months also showed no significant difference (.05 level of significance) between scores. Results did indicate, however, that overall performance levels of both verbal expression and expressive pantomime are significantly different (.05 level of

Table 5. *Planned comparisons of subgroups with analysis of variance*

Source	Df.	S.S.	M.S.	F.	P.	Multivariate F.	Df.	P.
Aphasics vs. Normals	–	——	——	——	——	41.02	2,34	.001
Sum	1	40960.00	40960.00	61.27	.0001	——	—	——
Difference	1	14288.40	14288.40	53.13	.0001	——	—	——
Normal Subgroups (By Age)	–	——	——	——	——	.7655	2,34	.473
Sum	1	984.25	984.25	1.47	.2372	——	—	——
Difference	1	4.65	4.65	.02	.8961	——	—	——
Aphasic Subgroups (by MPO)	–	——	——	——	——	1.2835	4,68	.2852
Sum	1	820.14	820.14	1.23	.3056	——	—	——
Difference	1	573.65	573.65	2.13	.1337	——	—	——
Error								
Sum	35	23399.95	668.57					
Difference	35	9413.25	268.95					

significance) between normal subjects and aphasic subjects, and the variation between verbal and pantomime subtest scores is also found to differ significantly for the two groups (ratio=41.02, degrees of freedom=2, 34).

Expressive pantomime was found to be superior to verbal expression for both normal and aphasic subjects as demonstrated by the mean scores in Table 2, with pantomime scoring 35 points higher than verbal expression for the aphasic group. The significant difference between verbal and pantomimic performances is thus found to favor expressive pantomime in aphasic subjects. The null hypothesis is, therefore, rejected in concluding that the aphasic patient is better able to use expressive pantomime than verbal expression in controlled communicative situations.

Discussion
Comparisons with prior research
Previous studies in the area of gesture and pantomime as related to aphasia have accumulated diverse and varying results. While Goodglass and Kaplan (1963) concluded from their research that aphasics demonstrate a gestural deficiency which is best understood as an apraxic disorder, they refute the concept that gestural deficiency implies a general communicative disorder. Pickett (1972) views the gestural impairment in aphasics as a part of the total communication

118

deficit rather than as a result of limb apraxia, while Duffy, Duffy and Pearson (1975) found aphasics poorer than normal subjects in pantomime recognition which they attributed to an underlying symbolic disorder evident in all modalities. Although the depressed scores achieved by the aphasic subjects within this study on both the verbal and pantomimic tasks suggest an overall impairment in communicative skills as a result of the aphasic syndrome, the distinct superiority of pantomime over verbal expression rejects the assertion of Duffy, Duffy and Pearson (1975) that an underlying symbolic disorder affects all modalities similarly.

Rather than investigating the gestural ability of aphasics as a function of overall communicative impairments in the symbolic process or according to specific levels of severity, intellectual functioning, or limb apraxia, this study chose to compare the intra-personal differences which exist between verbal expression and expressive pantomime in individual aphasic patients. The sole restriction from participation in the study was an inability to perform either task following training on pretest items. Data gathered from normal subjects provided an adequate baseline from which to judge the verbal and pantomimic performances of aphasics as compared to a general population; however, the purpose of the investigation was to examine each aphasic to determine which modality would facilitate the most effective communication. While age and months post onset of stroke exhibited no significant influence on performance ability, it appears evident that aphasic subjects were able to utilize expressive pantomime significantly better than verbal expression.

Explanation of the superior abilities with nonverbal communication through pantomime implies a need for further research in the area. If aphasia is actually a central symbolic disorder as Duffy, Duffy and Pearson (1975) concluded, both verbal and nonverbal communicative abilities would be affected; however, the findings of this study that pantomimic abilities exceed those of verbal expression indicate true potential in implementation of gesture and pantomime as an alternate mode of communication for the aphasic patient.

Therapeutic implications
Since the basic goal in working with an aphasic client in speech therapy lies in improving his ability to communicate his thoughts and ideas to other people, the therapist must stimulate expression

119

through any possible modality. An inherent strength in expressive pantomime would suggest implementation of gesture and pantomime for communication which would effectively circumvent the impaired oral verbal channel of the aphasic. Utilization of this nonverbal mode of communication may re-establish the bonds of human interaction while restoring the aphasic's self-concept and psychological well-being by demonstrating that his ability to think remains completely intact despite verbal deficits (Schlanger, 1976).

Contemporary authorities in the area of nonverbal communication suggest that gesture and pantomime may be executed more rapidly than speech to convey complex meanings effectively without syntactic or morphologic complications for the aphasic (Critchley, 1939; Alajouanine and Lhermitte, 1964). However, the most accurate communication is believed to occur when both verbal and nonverbal symbols are used simultaneously (Martin, 1962; Leathers, 1976).

Vocal overflow in expressive pantomime
Throughout this study, the phenomenon described by Goodglass and Kaplan (1963) as 'vocal overflow' presented itself in both normal and aphasic subjects. Verbal remarks were emitted accompanying the action which was being portrayed, apparently as a result of the subjects' inability to separate pantomimic movements from the immediate involvement in the movement itself. Even when the aphasic subjects were unable to produce adequate verbal expression, vocal sounds were frequently utilized as if to supplement or enhance the pretended action.

Although pantomime may not be employed as the aphasic's primary mode of communication, success with use of the nonverbal system may provide reinforcement for verbal attempts to communicate and act as a catalyst to promote more language output (Schlanger, 1976). The aphasic patient who has achieved higher levels of verbal output may also benefit from the incorporation of pantomime therapy as a retrieval cue for stimulating production of appropriate oral language.

Training in pantomime
Although pantomimic tasks elicited higher scores than verbal tasks for both groups of subjects, adaptation to the utilization of communicative movements without verbal output proved initially difficult

for all test subjects. Verbal subtest items required very little training prior to actual administration of the subtest, yet all four training items were frequently needed to effectively establish the target behavior which was desired for the pantomimic subtest. This may suggest an increased efficiency in the use of gesture and pantomime following implementation of training with a more specific program than the one used within this evaluative procedure.

Schlanger, Gaffner and DiCarrado (1974) conducted an experiment in training aphasics of various levels of severity to utilize pantomimic communication by eliciting the desired motor responses from aphasics solely through gestures using no verbal cues. Four subjects, two diagnosed as Group One aphasia and the other two diagnosed as Group Five aphasia according to the *Minnesota Test for Differential Diagnosis of Aphasia*, were evaluated for pantomimic performance both before a training period and following the training to assess improvement. The two subjects with good use of functional speech displayed better gestural ability at the onset than the two subjects who had no functional speech; however, even the group without speech showed marked improvement after training. Such findings lead investigators to the assumption that even individuals with severe aphasic involvements may profit from pantomimic instruction in both receptive and expressive language skills.

Direction for further research
Expressive pantomime is one mode of communication which may prove extremely valuable in therapeutic application with the aphasic patient. When employed to elicit or enhance meaningful communication of mildly to severely impaired aphasic patients, it appears that gestural communication holds great potential for circumventing linguistic deficits. Further research is needed, particularly in the area of training aphasics with pantomimic communication, so that documentation may specify successful training techniques, the effectiveness of training larger groups of aphasics, the time period during recovery which is most beneficial for beginning pantomime training, and the instruction which is required by those people around the aphasic patient so that they may interpret his intended meaning. Additional investigation is vital to establish the effectiveness of pantomimic communication with documented results, yet the strength of pantomimic expression over verbal expression suggests true potential

in pantomime as one avenue of approach for therapy with the aphasic client.

Summary and conclusion
The present investigation was undertaken in an attempt to assess oral verbal expression and the pantomime abilities of aphasic patients to determine if the two modes of communication are equally impaired.

Twenty normal subjects and twenty aphasic subjects were evaluated within both communicative modes. Normal subjects selected from a random population were divided into two age groups ranging from 20 to 49 years and from 50 to 80 years. Subjects classified as demonstrating aphasic symptoms ranged in age from 58 to 83 years and were selected from four convalescent centers in northeastern and east central Indiana. Following the administration and adequate performance on four training items from each subtest, a series of ten colored drawings picturing common objects was shown to each subject under two conditions. With presentation proceeding in random order, each subject identified the function of the pictured items both verbally and through the use of pantomime. Responses were then scored according to the PICA multidimensional binary choice system.

After establishing reliability and internal consistency for the testing procedure through computation of Crombach's Alpha, data was interpreted by means of multivariate and univariate analysis of variance. Planned comparisons indicated that there was no significant difference between groups according to age or months post onset of stroke; however, the overall performance and the variation between subtest scores was significant between aphasic and normal subjects at the .05 level of significance. Mean scores indicated that both normal and aphasic subjects performed more effectively through use of pantomime than verbal expression although the mean difference for aphasics was 35 points while the normal subjects had a mean difference of only 1 point between the two modalities. The null hypothesis was rejected to establish that performance through expressive pantomime is superior to that of oral verbal expression in aphasic patients.

Current research indicates a significance in the implementation of gesture and expressive pantomime with aphasics which aphasiologists have only recently begun to consider. Further studies in the area of nonverbal communication deficits in aphasia are needed to establish a fuller understanding of the nature of aphasia as well as to supplement possibilities for implementing pantomimic expression in the training program of the aphasic patient.

5

PROSODIC ASPECTS IN THE RECEPTION OF LANGUAGE*

GILBERT ASSAL, JOCELYNE BUTTET, ERIC ZANDER

Introduction

The neuropsychological approach to aphasia constitutes a method by which to consider more effective measures of treatment and to stimulate interest in the value of reeducation. Often aphasics, during the course of their therapy, show more progress than the classical tests predict. This disagreement is disturbing for the observer, particularly since the relatives of and therapists with aphasic patients can give examples which leave no doubt about the degree of improvement. Our hypothesis, which has been developed on the basis of clinical observations, is that many aphasics become gradually better able to use suprasegmental cues, of which we think prosody is the most important.

Prosody has long been the true neglected child of linguistics and has been considered only marginally. During the past few years, however, language specialists have become aware of its considerable scope; they have recaptured the conception of Aristotle (1969) that speech is the symbol of the mind.

In comparing propositional language to emotional language Jackson (1932) included inflections of the voice in the latter. He also attributed the function of emotional and automatic language to the right hemisphere. However, emotions are far from being just automatic processes; for example, the inflections of the voice in the aphasic patient are not only used in the involuntary expression of emotions, but also to participate in the deliberate communication of feelings and intentions.

In aphasiology and in neuropsychology the concept of prosody evokes the name of Monrad-Krohn (1947) who introduced the term

* Swiss National Science Foundation No 3,2450.74.

dysprosody. In the studies of the Norwegian neurologist, three aspects of prosody are stressed: prosody is intrinsic to language; it is propositional; it is emotional. Moreover, Monrad-Krohn insists on the considerable variations of prosody between individuals and between subjects of different races.

These references to Jackson and to Monrad-Kohn indicate our frame of research using a clinical basis. In our study we seek to define a possible deficit in cases of lesions of the cerebral cortex and to describe this impairment in relation to functional localization.

In the following paragraphs, we refer to an analogy between recognition of faces and that of voices. The disorder defined by Bodamer (1947) as *prosopagnosia* has been isolated, described and correlated with bilateral damage to the posterior lobes, predominantly on the right side. This work was independent of research in experimental psychology; neither the procedures nor the eventual invariants in the recognition of faces were taken into account. We proceeded with the same perspective in our study of voices. Some will recognize in this approach the influence of our teacher Hécaen, who has contributed to our knowledge in this domain, along with the work of Tzavaras (1967), which he inspired. During the first stages of our study (which this work presents) we deliberately have neglected the psychophysical element.

Recognition of voice and prosody
One of the first questions has to do with the role of prosody in the recognition of voices. Some linguists, such as Fónagy (1976), point out that when an expressive particularity occurs repeatedly in the pronunciation of an individual, it acquires an identifying function. The pertinent question, in the case of the recognition of voices, is to distinguish variable from constant features in each individual.

Darwin (1975) indicates that it is prosody which makes continual perception of speech possible. This process depends upon the identification of the voice of the speaker. It enables one to isolate one voice among many, as in a cocktail party. We will return to this subject when we discuss the work of Darwin.

The recognition of human voices begins early in the new-born. Mehler *et al.* (1976) have shown that as early as one month, a baby is able to identify his mother's voice as long as she is addressing him with her usual intonation. Suppression of melody (monopitch) abolishes this recognition. Distortion of the voice by a filter also greatly disturbs the identification. Numerous studies have been done with infants to determine their reactions to a voice and particularly to the mother's voice; these studies underline the interest the child has for the voice of his mother in comparison with other auditory stimuli he receives (Friedlander, 1968).

In another study which is similar to our own, Mann et al. (1977) have dealt with voice recognition in school age children. In the first stages, this group followed the same pattern as in the development of recognition of familiar and unfamiliar faces by the child (Carey et al., 1977; Diamond et al., 1977). In their study, Mann et al. have presented sentences composed of six syllables spoken by six young women unknown to the child. The sentences were given in pairs, where four possibilities were represented: the same voice – same or different sentences; different voices – same or different sentences. The child had to indicate if he heard one or two speakers. At the age of six, which was the youngest group tested, the level of performance was just above chance. At the age of ten, in the condition where the sentences were identical, the discrimination of voices by the child reached the same level of success as observed in the adult subject. However, this is not the case when different sentences were given. The authors conclude that the curves of acquisition of face recognition and voice recognition are parallel.

In the adult, there is considerable capability to recognize voices. Pollak et al. (1954) emphasized this fact in their study where subjects were able to identify a speaker with a high percentage of correct responses. This identification was made among sixty-five familiar voices and after hearing only a few words. The identification of voices has also been the subject of multiple studies by espionage services and the police. The results underscore the accuracy and the consistency of the identification of speakers on the basis of hearing their voices.

The acoustic characteristics of speech give us some information about the identity of the speaker, including biological features, such as age and sex, as well as socio-cultural features. They inform us also about his affective state and his motivations.

Affective or emotional intonations are distinguished from linguistic intonations. This dichotomy, already cited by Monrad-Krohn, is generally accepted by linguists (Delattre, 1966). It is relatively easy

127

to categorize the various linguistic intonations, but it is difficult to classify emotional intonations. The presence of an emotion is easily acknowledged, but its interpretation varies widely from one listener to the next. Also, there exists a whole range of nuances. For example, interrogation can have different forms: simple, which is generally accepted as having no affective connotation, incredulous, or astonished.

The recognition of emotional intonations varies according to the particular nature of the intonation. For instance, anger is generally easily identifiable. The type of information and the conditions in which it is delivered to the listener are also to be taken into account. Indeed, these factors induce certain modes of intonation.

As was previously noted, intonation is an important factor in the perception of the continuity of speech. This is explained well in a study by Darwin (1975). In dichotic conditions, the subject hears with each ear words spoken by one speaker; he has to carry out the task of shadowing (simultaneous repetition) the message delivered to one ear and he must not alternate in this task from one ear to the other. The shifting of the semantic continuity from one ear to the other does not disturb the task. On the contrary, if it is the intonation which is shifted, the subject finds himself repeating what is received by the ear he was instructed to neglect.

Prosodic continuity also plays a role in the capability to retain verbal sequences and to understand them. In this respect we will mention especially studies introducing conflicts between syntax and prosody (Wingfield et al., 1971; Wingfield, 1975). Intelligibility diminishes when the prosodic boundary occurs before the syntactic boundary; if this process is reversed, one finds no disturbances when the sentences are presented at a normal speed. However, when the sentences are compressed in time, without modifying the pitch, an increase of the verbal flow (compression) impairs intelligibility in a continuous and progressive way in the sentences where syntax and prosody are in conflict. When there is no conflict, intelligibility remains good until a certain compression rate is reached, where it breaks down.

Furthermore, sentences composed of isolated concatenated (without intonation) words can be totally incomprehensible.

In dichotic listening, a slight left ear superiority obtains for the recognition of non-verbal emotional stimuli such as laughing, shouting, and sighing (King and Kimura, 1972; Carmon and Nachson, 1973). Identical acoustic information can be better processed by the left hemisphere in a linguistic context, and by the right hemisphere if it is presented as a purely acoustic task. Using the dichotic listening procedure, Van Lancker and Fromkin (1973) found a difference between speakers of Thai (a tone language) and English speakers. When pitch differences occurred within language stimuli, the Thai speakers demonstrated a right ear superiority whereas these same subjects did not show such an asymmetry for pitch differences alone (hums). Results with English-speaking subjects failed to show a difference between these two types of stimuli. This study led the authors to conclude that pitch discrimination is lateralized to the left hemisphere when the pitch differences are linguistically processed.

Cherry (1953) has shown that if a subject is engaged in a task of shadowing for material delivered at one ear, he does not easily perceive changes in verbal material occurring at the other ear, for example, a change of language (shifting from English to German). On the other hand, he has no difficulty in differentiating speakers of different sexes. Since the task of shadowing undoubtedly involves the left hemisphere, one may assume that the acoustic discrimination of sex is a function of the right hemisphere. On the other hand, Doehring and Ross (1972) have found a slight right ear superiority when the subject is required to indicate which of three voices, speaking a nonsense syllable (consonant–vowel–consonant), matches the speaker of a sample vowel.

In another experiment, Doehring and Bartholomeus (1971) presented a sample voice binaurally; the subject was required to indicate which of two dichotically-presented voices matched the sample voice. Three different kinds of stimuli were used. Twice, a significant right ear superiority was found. In another study, Bartholomeus (1971) presented a series of dichotic trials, each involving two different sequences of letters sung to two different melodies by two different singers. Three tasks were required: to repeat the letters, to reproduce the melodies or to recognize the voices. Results indicated significant right ear superiority for letter sequence recognition, significant left ear superiority for melody recognition, but no significant difference between ears in recognition of sung voices.

Studies devoted to the recognition of emotions in dichotic listening can be divided into two groups. In the first group, the task consists in

129

recognizing an intonation whose nature is emotional or linguistic. The recognition is considered in itself and does not imply any linguistic decision as to the verbal material which supports it, since a filter is used to suppress all intelligibility. In this condition, Blumstein and Cooper (1974) have demonstrated a left ear superiority for the identification of different linguistic intonations. This advantage obtains whether the subjects have to identify the intonation by naming the corresponding sentence type or by pointing to the appropriate sketched contour pattern. Using natural sentences in an emotional tone, Haggard and Parkinson (1971) also found a left ear advantage for this kind of identification.

The second group of studies reveal a right ear superiority for verbal material involving an intonation. However, in these tasks the intonation does not have to be recognized or identified. For example, verbal material made of nonsense syllables, structured as in an English sentence, needs the presence of intonation to be better perceived in the right than in the left ear by English-speaking listeners (Zurif *et al.*, 1970 and 1972). In the same vein, the illusion that consists in shifting the unexpected arrival of a click on a syntactic boundary shows a right ear superiority when the sentences are intonated (Clark quoted by Zurif, 1974).

Agnosia for prosody
A pathology of the recognition of prosody has never been described. Neither have difficulties in the identification of speakers using the auditory modality been reported, apart from epileptical verbal hallucinations with lack of recognition of the speaker or of his emotional state (Hécaen and Ajuriaguerra, 1964). As a matter of fact, an alteration of voice quality was noticed by Dordain *et al.* (1971) in right brain damaged patients. The authors found modifications of the register of the voice and of the rate of speech in many left hemiplegics, some of whom had great trouble varying the intensity of their speech.

In spite of the misgivings of Monrad-Krohn (1947), it is difficult not to refer to the pathology of musical abilities. Assal *et al.* (1973, 1977) observed aphasic musicians in whom musical skills were still very high, or even intact. They also described a professional violinist, who had a severe disturbance in musical expression and recognition following a fronto-temporal right hemispheric lesion. This obser-

130

vation is very similar to that reported by Botez and Wertheim (1959).

In a series of more systematic studies, Milner (1962) demonstrated that after right but not after left temporal lobectomies, patients present a decreased capacity for recognizing timbre of voices as well as diminution of tonal memory.

Using the Wada technique, Bogen and Gorden (1971) showed that after sodium amytal injection in the right carotid, there are only slight modifications of speech, while singing is very severely impaired, especially in its melodic aspect. We have been able to verify this during an epileptic seizure in a patient with a right frontal lesion.

Starting with Brissaud (1894, 1901), aphasiologists have discussed only disturbances in the production of prosody. Pick (1913) discussed an alteration of prosody in agrammatism. Monrad-Krohn (1947) described dysprosody in an aphasic Norwegian woman whose expression involved a German accent. The disorder disappeared when she was singing. Monrad-Krohn insisted on the distinction between prosody and music and rejected expressions such as the *song* or *the melody of language*.

More recently, Goodglass *et al.* (1967) reconsidered the problem of prosody in agrammatic patients. They underscored the difficulty these patients have in initiating a sentence with an unstressed word.

In split-brain subjects the reproduction of brief melodies presented dichotically does not show any superiority of the right hemisphere, perhaps because this hemisphere alone is not able to assume control of the vocal musculature effectively (Milner, 1974). However, the role of the right hemisphere in musical activities seems to be widely confirmed by the studies with split-brain patients conducted by Franco (1977). In a reading task, which activates the left hemisphere, a concomitant elaborated activity is possible only with the left hand. On the contrary, in a musical task, only the right hand can perform well with the same type of activity.

Taub *et al.* (1976) have discovered differences in evoked potentials, indicating a preponderance of the right hemisphere for nonverbal auditory stimuli such as musical chords.

Neither musical recognition nor musical expression in their multiple aspects need to be the exclusive property of one single hemisphere. Using the dichotic procedure, a tonal superiority for the right ear and a left ear advantage for timbre have been shown (Charbonneau &

131

Risset, 1975). Furthermore, the level of musical training, probably because of the use of different strategies after training, is a very important factor (Bever & Chiarello, 1974).

The problem of the relationships between recognition of voices and intonations and recognition of faces and mimics has been raised several times. Some authors assert that the recognition of voices can compensate for a deficit in the identification of faces, but such a generalization seems to be unfounded. Patients' claims that they are able to recognize voices is no guarantee that this aptitude is actually preserved. Indeed, their identification may be based entirely on the speaker's style of speech. Moreover, a review of some observations of prosopagnosics teaches us that the voice is not a constant aid for identification (Hécaen and Angelergues, 1963; Tzavaras, 1967).

On the basis of fairly limited material, Grenier (1969) compared performances on recognition tasks with regard to the side of the lesion. She found more severe difficulties in the recognition of voices than of faces in the event of right hemispheric lesions. On the other hand, Green and Boller (1974) demonstrated that in spite of severe auditory comprehension deficits, aphasics retain the ability to distinguish between certain modalities of intonation (interrogative versus delarative, etc.). Blumstein and Goodglass (1972) showed that aphasics, notwithstanding their handicap, can recognize and utilize stress, which permits lexical differentiation in the English language. In twelve subjects with temporoparietal lesions, six on the right side and six on the left, Heilman et al. (1975) studied the recognition of affective intonations and the recognition of sentence meaning. Identification of the meaning of the sentences did not cause any problem in the population studied. On the other hand, the recognition of intonations was impaired in both groups of patients, but significantly more so with right lesions than with left lesions, whatever the modality of the response. The subjects answered either by pointing to the picture of a face, the expression of which was judged to correspond to the voice heard, or by naming orally the corresponding emotion. The authors regard this deficit more as an impairment in the discrimination of emotions than as a problem of auditory discrimination.

Schlanger et al. (1976) studied the capacities of unilateral brain-damaged subjects for the recognition of three different emotions in semantic and asemantic sentences. Subjects had to respond by pointing to the picture of the face judged to correspond to the intonation. The poorest results were obtained with severe aphasics, followed by the patients with right-sided lesions and finally the moderate aphasics. A significant difference was found only between the high- and the low-verbal aphasics.

Personal studies

We mentioned in an earlier presentation (Assal *et al.*, 1972) that patients with right hemispheric lesions had more difficulties in recognizing emotional and linguistic intonations than did patients with left lesions. Moreover, we cited a positive correlation between the lack of ability to identify these intonations and an inability to discriminate between two voices, either the same or two different voices, in a task where two semantic or asemantic sentences were presented. However, in the intonation task, the response was made by choosing from among six drawings expressing, in a caricatured manner, anger, sadness, interrogation, etc. Therefore, errors made by right brain damaged patients may have been due, at least in part, to a prosopagnosic or visuospatial disorder. As for the aphasics, we found the relatively complicated procedure an obstacle in that the task required them to explain the different intonations and to indicate which one matched the faces. Because of these various factors, which could not be adequately controlled, the value of our findings is limited.

In another study (Assal *et al.*, 1976) we restricted ourselves to studying the recognition of the voices of speakers. In the first stage of our research, we compared the performances of 29 control subjects (CS) and 47 patients, 22 with left hemisphcric lesions (LL) and 25 with right hemispheric lesions (RL). The two groups of patients do not significantly differ in their etiology or in the severity of their neurological deficits.

The test consisted of pairs of short French sentences such as *Tu as soif* (you are thirsty) or *Il a faim* (he is hungry) spoken by one or two different speakers. The response – 'there is one voice' or 'there are two voices' – was made verbally or by pointing to a sign. Four possibilities were then proposed to the subject: the sentence is the same and the speaker is the same or there are two different speakers; the sentences are different and there are one or two speakers. Three subtests, each consisting of thirty pairs of sentences were presented. In the first test, there were six speakers (women, men and children) from the same geographic area. In the second test, there were five women originating from different countries (Germany, Great Britain, etc.). In the third test, there were five women from the same geographic area.

The patients, particularly those with right lesions, did understand and could use effectively the notion of sameness or difference. On a similar, but strictly linguistic task, the patients with right hemispheric lesions achieved normal scores.

Table 1. *Discrimination of voices*

Mean errors per group for all 3 tests

CS	N=29	13.7
LL	N=22	23.4
RL	N=25	28.1

The differences between CS and LL and between CS and RL are significant (Tuckey's test).

Table 1 indicates the results for all three tests. There is a significant difference between the group of control subjects and the group of left hemispheric lesion patients, and also between the controls and the right brain damaged patients. The right-sided lesion patients made more mistakes than the other two groups. However, their results do not significantly differ from the results of the left hemispheric lesion group.

Table 2. *Discrimination of voices*

Mean errors per group for each of the 3 tests

		Test 1	Test 2	Test 3
CS	N=29	2.9	5.5	5.3
		NS	*	*
LL	N=22	3.8	8.5	11.1
		NS	*	NS
RL	N=25	4.7	10.8	12.6
		*	*	*
CS	N=29	2.9	5.5	5.3

* Significant difference (Tuckey's test).

Table 2 shows the results for each of the three tests. In the first test, a significant difference exists only between the control subjects and the group with right lesions. In the second test, significant differences are found between the control group and the group with left lesions,

134

the control group and the group with right lesions, and also between the two groups of brain-damaged patients. In the third test, significant differences are observed between the control group and the group with right lesions and between the control group and the group with left lesions, but the difference between the patients with left- and right-sided lesions does not reach a significant level.

Table 3. *Discrimination of voices—Patients with left hemisphere lesions*

Mean errors per sub-group as a function of presence or absence of aphasia

	Test 1	Test 2	Test 3	Sum of all 3 tests
Aphasic patients	3.8	9.2	11.6	24.5
N=17	NS	NS	NS	NS
Non-aphasic patients	3.8	6.2	9.6	19.6
N=5				

NS=not significant ('t' test)

A high percentage of patients in the LL group presented language disorders in the broadest sense. The results of these patients do not differ from those of the LL patients without aphasic problems, however (see Table 3). Considering only disorders of auditory comprehension, which were present in 64 per cent of the left cerebral lesions, we find that this group of patients had difficulty in voice discrimination, but their results do not differ significantly from those of patients with normal comprehension (see Table 4).

Table 4. *Discrimination of voices—Patients with left hemisphere lesions*

Mean errors per sub-group as a function of presence or absence of auditory comprehension disorders

	Test 1	Test 2	Test 3	Sum of all 3 tests
Deficits in comprehension	3.7	8.9	10.8	23.4
N=14	NS	NS	NS	NS
Normal comprehension	3.8	7.8	11.8	23.4
N=8				

NS=not significant ('t' test)

In the dichotic listening test for verbal material we found a noticeable percentage (32%) of patients with right cerebral lesions suffering

135

from relative or absolute extinction of the left ear. If we compare the two groups of patients (with and without extinction in the dichotic test), we find that this parameter is significant. The results of the patients with extinction of the left ear are always the poorest, at a significant level, except in the first test (see Table 5).

Table 5. *Discrimination of voices—Patients with right hemisphere lesions*

Mean errors per sub-group as a function of presence or absence of extinction in the dichotic listening test

	Test 1	Test 2	Test 3	Sum of all 3 tests
Presence of extinction	5.4	14.5	16	35.9
N=8	NS	**	**	*
Absence of extinction	4.4	9.1	11	24.5
N=17				

*p<.05 ('t' test)   **p<.01 ('t' test)

When the voices are acoustically similar, i.e. two childish voices, two female or two male voices, the means of errors of the control subjects (2.2), of the left lesion group (2.9), and of the right lesion group (2.8) do not differ significantly. When the voices are relatively similar, i.e. one voice of a woman and one voice of a child, there is a distinct difference: the control subjects and the patients with left hemispheric lesions perform at the same level (0.1 and 0.3 errors respectively) whereas the subjects with right hemispheric lesions have more errors (1.2). In cases where the acoustic difference is more striking, one voice of a man and one voice of a child, errors are not made by the control subjects nor the left hemispheric lesion patients. On the other hand, four patients with right hemispheric lesions (16%) made errors on this task.

In a third study, we asked a revision of the tests described above. These new tests of discrimination gave results which are comparable in all respects to the previous data (see Table 6). We also subjected the patients to a forced-choice procedure, based on the work of Carey for face recognition (1977). In these tasks, we introduced an added difficulty in the discrimination of voices by altering either the context or the prosodic elements. The characteristics of context used to help elicit the desired response or to induce a false choice included

136

Table 6. *Discrimination of voices* (*new version*)

Mean errors per group

	Test 1	Test 2	Test 3	Sum of all 3 tests
CS N=33	3.3	10.3	6.4	20
LL N=22	4.9	13.6	10.3	28.8
RL N=20	7.4	16.2	12.6	37.2

Test 1 = 5 French-speaking speakers (1 man, 2 women, 2 children)
Test 2 = 5 women with foreign accents
Test 3 = 5 women speaking Hebrew

sentences or liaisons (sounding of final consonant before initial vowel sound), regional prosodic characteristics, foreign accents, and emotional intonations. A third of the items implied a true choice, since there was no conflict between the paraphernalia added to the model and those present in the multiple choices. The data from this study remained fragmentary, due to the limited number of patients.

Analyzing the results, incomplete as they may be, we find that two distinct situations are seen depending upon the two variables:
series A: sentences and liaisons
series B: imitated regional and foreign accents and emotional
  intonations.

Table 7. *Paraphernalia—Series A*

Mean errors per group

	Sentences	Liaisons
CS N=33	5.4	3.5
LL N=16	6.8	8
RL N=13	6.6	7.6

Generally speaking, performances of the patients with right cerebral lesions are inferior to those of patients with left cerebral lesions. A particularly great difference is observed when we compare the first series of tests –A– to the second series –B–. For the first series (see Table 7), the results are slightly better in cases of right than of left cerebral lesions, whereas for the second series of tests, left cerebral lesion patients scored higher (see Table 8). In the test using foreign accents, we find that the control subjects and the left hemispheric patients are at the same level, whereas the right brain damaged patients are clearly inferior.

Table 8. *Paraphernalia—Series B*

Mean errors per group

		Intonations	Foreign Accents	Regional Accents
CS	N=33	8	7.6	8.6
LL	N=16	10.4	7.6	9.4
RL	N=13	11.2	9.6	10

We consider the difficulties with voice recognition seen in cases of right cerebral damage to be a definite entity. These difficulties have been found three times in successive studies whose common characteristics are quite obvious. Moreover, the studies have been performed with three different samples of patients. A similar profile of performance is found no matter whether the modality of response is a judgment of 'same–different' or a match. The same pattern of errors in cases of unilateral hemispheric lesions (right yielding more errors than left) has also been found in another series of studies which we have not mentioned. One of these studies consisted of sentences where a possible change of speakers occurs either at a syntactic boundary or within a syntactic unit. Another task required recognition of familiar voices from amidst unfamiliar voices. A third study tested normal subjects on a task of dichotic voice recognition. The results showed a left ear superiority with all test materials utilizing short sentences.

In the two test series mentioned above (A and B), the deficits appeared more or less selective as a function of the characteristics of each test. When the acoustic differences were small, the task became too difficult even for the control group. On the contrary, with testing variables such as accents and intonations, a clear separation occurred between the control and the brain-damaged subjects and also between the patients with differing hemispheric lesions. We found that patients with right hemispheric lesions were frequently successful in simple voice identification, as when French-speaking voices were presented without the complication of different intonations or accents. This suggests that the left hemisphere has some influence in this function of simple identification. On the other hand, when the invariant pertaining to voice must be extracted from more complex test material, the task demands the intervention of the right hemisphere.

The recognition of voices may be effected independently of the comprehension of speech, as the results from sensory aphasics reveal. Both the control subjects and the patients give better results with sentences spoken in an unknown language; the subjects benefit perhaps from the absence of interference related to language context.

Conclusions

Our results support the view, already put forward in early descriptions of aphasia, that some attributes of speech can correctly be identified even in cases of word-deafness. However, such ability is not always preserved in left brain damaged patients.

Regarding voice identification, our results indicate that the right hemisphere plays an important part. This is at variance with Doehring and colleagues' conclusion (1972) that in normal subjects the left hemisphere is more important than the right in the identification of voice. The disagreement may be due to the difference in the test materials used. As a matter of fact, our findings tend to show that both hemispheres play a part in speaker recognition; it is possible that in this task each half of the brain uses a different strategy, however. Under difficult identification circumstances, the right hemisphere appears to play the more important part. It is also dominant when the left hemisphere is dealing with some other task. This difference of functions between the two hemispheres is one of the most difficult problems in neuropsychology. Where is the information finally synthetized that has been analyzed by different neuronal circuits?

This theoretical problem is very important for speech therapists who know very well the help that melodic support can provide in severe problems of expression; the often remarkable results of melodic intonation therapy show such assistance (Albert *et al.*, 1973). To what measure can an intact function, which shares certain neuronic elements with an altered function, contribute to the process of restoration of the impaired function?

If it is true that the right hemisphere plays a leading part in voice recognition as it does in face recognition, then this hemisphere may be considered dominant for the recognition of human individuality. This conclusion would accord with hypotheses formulated by Hécaen, who considers that the right hemisphere is dominant for tasks of individualization within categories. When this hemisphere is severely disturbed, there may be a real social agnosia (Kling, 1972).

139

6

DYSCALCULIA IN A RIGHT-HANDED TEACHER OF MATHEMATICS WITH RIGHT CEREBRAL DAMAGE

CHANTAL LELEUX, GUDRUN KAISER, YVAN LEBRUN

Acalculia is a descriptive term used originally by Henschen (1920) to denote an acquired disorder of calculation. Apparently, no case of pure acalculia has ever been reported and a computational defect is always mentioned as one of several neuropsychological symptoms, generally associated with aphasia. In the available literature, most cases of acalculia are due to a left hemispheric lesion or result from bilateral brain disease (e.g. Lewandowsky and Stadelmann, 1908; Peritz, 1918; Sittig, 1921; Berger, 1926; Singer and Low, 1933; Lindqvist, 1935, 1936; Benson and Weir, 1972).

At the end of the 19th century and at the beginning of the 20th century it was assumed that in right-handed subjects the left hemisphere was dominant for all symbolic functions. Consequently, this was generally held to be the only part of the brain concerned with calculation. According to Peritz (1918): 'Rechenstörung bei Hinterhauptsverletzten findet sich nur dann, wenn die linke Gehirnhälfte getroffen ist; bei rechtsseitigen Verletzungen ist die Rechenfähigkeit stets eine gute (...). In der Gegend des linken Gyrus angularis scheint ein Zentrum für das Rechnen zu liegen.' Berger (1926) maintained 'dass die linke Hemisphäre beim Rechtshänder stets betroffen gefunden wurde, wenn es zu Rechenstörungen kam (...). Von der linken Hemisphäre war nun vorwiegend betroffen der Occipitallappen (...) Sicherlich ist aber auch der linke Temporallappen an dem Zustandekommen der Rechenstörungen beteiligt.' Henschen (1927) also claimed that 'die Rechenfähigkeit sich zur linken Hemisphäre begrenzt.' More recently, Sperry et al. (1969), reporting on commissurotomized subjects, stated that 'tests for mathematical performance in the minor hemisphere with nonverbal readout and with the sensory

141

input restricted to the left visual field or the left hand indicate that the capacity for calculation on the minor side is almost negligible. By manipulating marbles or dowel sticks, watching spots of light flashed to the left field and pointing with the left hand, these patients may succeed in matching numbers or in adding one to numbers below ten but they fail when required to add or subtract two or higher numbers and they fail also at the simplest tasks in multiplication and division.' Sperry *et al.* conclude accordingly that calculation is organized predominantly in the major hemisphere.*

However, as far back as 1886, Oppenheim (quoted by Lindqvist, 1935) seems to have laid stress on the relative independence of language and calculation and to have pointed out that reckoning abilities depend partly on the right hemisphere. In 1908 (p. 843) he briefly mentioned a patient with left hemiplegia and dyscalculia.

Oppenheim's opinion was dissonant from the views generally held by his contemporaries and by the next generation of aphasiologists, who regarded the left hemisphere as dominant for language as well as for calculation. At most, the right hemisphere was considered capable of elementary computations, when the left half of the brain had suffered some damage. Henschen (1926) thought that 'in calculation the visual factor plays an important role and the left hemisphere is generally the more concerned with it. It is not impossible that in some cases the right hemisphere can act as a substitute for the left when this is severely damaged, at least in simple counting and enumeration of figures. The enumeration of figures becomes by training a mechanical or automatic process, and it is probably for this reason that the right hemisphere is able to act as a substitute.' Goldstein (1948, p. 136) expressed a similar view: 'Performance gained by the other hemisphere may, in defects of the dominant one, help calculation by the support through visual or motor patterns.' Goldstein also stated that 'disturbances of calculation are more frequent in lesion of the dominant hemisphere than of the minor, probably because for the intellectual ability underlying calculation the dominant hemisphere is of greater importance.'

Critchley (1953) seems to agree with this. Disease of the dominant hemisphere, he believes, is more often followed by severe disorders of calculation than disease of the non-dominant half of the brain.

However, Kleist in 1934 (p. 563) remarked on 'die nicht seltenen Rechenstörungen bei rechts-verletzten Rechtsern.' And Cohen in

* This conclusion is qualified in an addendum to the paper, however.

1961 insisted that calculation disorder is by no means rare in right-handed patients with unilateral right brain damage.

Collignon *et al.* (1977), examining the correlation between calculation disorders and the side of the lesion, found a slightly higher frequency of the disturbances following left-sided pathology, but the difference did not exceed 5%.

Nowadays, there is general agreement that a lesion in the right hemisphere may easily entail visuo-spatial dyscalculia, e.g. computational difficulties due mainly to left visual neglect and to misplacement of the figures (e.g. Hécaen *et al.*, 1961; Héceaen, 1962, 1969; Ullmann, 1974). This is consonant with the attested superiority of the right hemisphere in visuo-spatial tasks and with Franco and Sperry's findings (1977) that in commissurotomized and in hemispherectomized patients the right hemisphere shows a constant superiority for geometrical discrimination.

In addition, Hécaen *et al.* (1961) have observed that a right lesion can also entail genuine *anarithmetia*, i.e. true loss of computational abilities. This observation has been confirmed by Bresson *et al.* (1972) and Collignon *et al.* (1977).

In the following we report the case of a 40 year old right-handed teacher of mathematics, who demonstrated anarithmetia following unilateral right brain damage.

On November 1, 1978, J.P.L. was taken to hospital because of a sudden left-sided hemiplegia and dysarthria which had appeared during the night. Important events in his medical past history included two epileptic fits; the last had occurred three weeks before admission. No sign of hypertension was known.

Clinical examination showed a complete left hemiplegia accompanied by an inferior facial paralysis, and a deviation of the eyes to the right. The next day the patient was referred to the neurosurgical department (Prof. Dr. J. Brihaye) for further investigation. In addition to the left hemiplegia the examining neurologist found a deficit in all sensory modalities over the left side of the body. The CT scan evidenced a large fronto-parietal haematoma in the right hemisphere. This was confirmed by the arteriogram which demonstrated a displacement of the anterior cerebral artery to the left, but no vascular malformation was visible. The EEG showed anomalies over the right hemisphere, particularly in the temporal lobe.

During the next few days, the patient, who was rather slow and sleepy, received dexamethasone and his wakefulness improved significantly. On November 13, a craniotomy was performed and the haematoma, lying deep in the right fronto-parietal area, was evacuated. Post-operatively, the patient's condition was quite satisfactory and two weeks later he was sent to a rehabilitation centre. The motor deficit showed signs of recovery, mainly in the inferior limb, although a Babinski sign could still be elicited on the left, and the deep tendon reflexes remained exaggerated; there was still a sensory loss.

On November 6, a neurolinguistic examination of the patient had taken place. It was found that he was awake, well oriented in time and space and willing to co-operate, but he became fatigued very easily. There was some emotional lability.

Comprehension of oral language was unimpaired. The patient was rather talkative. Spontaneous speech and answers to questions were correct but dysarthric, articulation being impeded by the unilateral facial paralysis. Metalinguistic tests requiring application of grammatical transformations indicated that the patient had no difficulty shifting from one pattern of transformation to the other. He could also form sentences containing words given by the examiner.

On the other hand, as Fig. 1 shows, writing exhibited numerous reduplications of strokes and letters, additions of zeros in high numbers written under dictation, a slightly oblique orientation of the lines and a tendency to write only on the right side of the sheet of paper (though there was no hemianopia). When reading over what he had written, the patient failed to notice his mistakes and he had difficulty finding similar reduplications in a text written by the examiner. When reading, the patient could not easily pass from one line to the other and he showed a slight tendency to neglect the left part of the lines. This rather typical symptomatology pointed to a lesion in the right hemisphere.

Spatiotactile sensation was unimpaired in the right hand; on the left side, testing was precluded by the sensory loss.

Drawing was rather ill-structured and sometimes incomplete on the left side (Fig. 2). A spatial dyscalculia was observed due to the incorrect positioning of figures and numbers (Fig. 3). Moreover, there existed a concomitant genuine dyscalculia (=*anarithmetia*) affecting the mental performance of elementary operations.

There was no left hemiasomatognosia.

The test of Rey, which requires the patient to memorize a series of

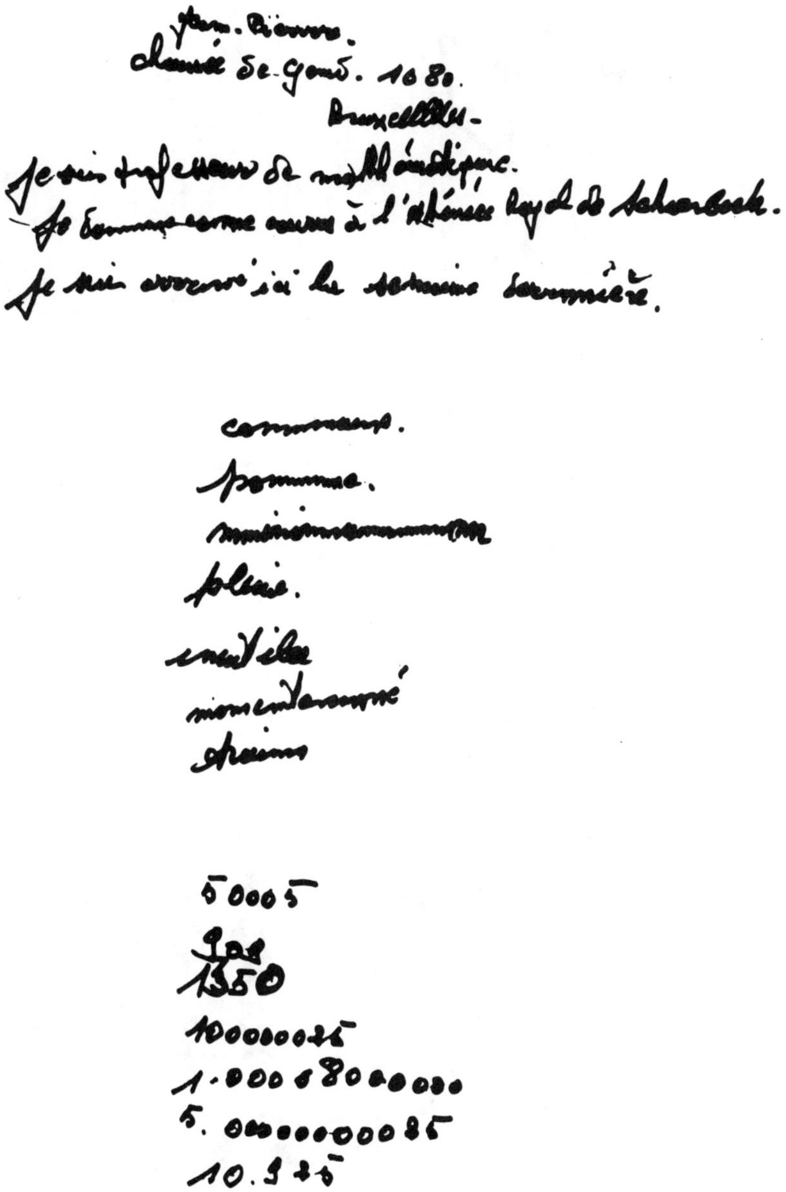

Figure 1

isolated words read out several times by the examiner, revealed an impairment of verbal short-term memory.

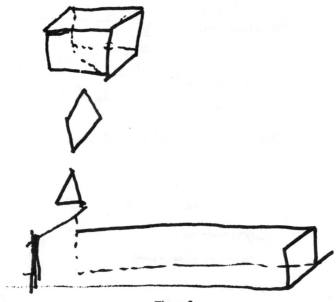

Figure 2

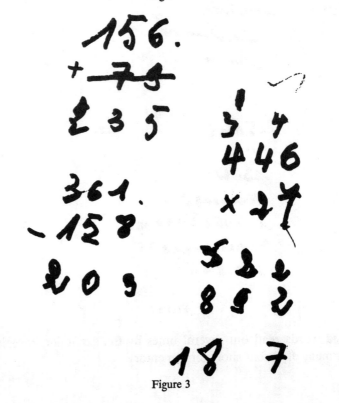

Figure 3

146

The patient was re-examined on November 20. Although a moderate afferent dysgraphia persisted, writing had improved significantly in comparison with the pre-operative examination. No neglect of the left side of the sheet was noticed and the discovery of superfluous strokes and letters in a text was almost normal. Reading was now correct and easy. Drawing was virtually normal.

In spite of this distinct improvement in most tasks, dyscalculia was still present, affecting mental and written calculation (Fig. 4). It appeared to result from a true disturbance of the computing mechanisms, since the visuospatial disorder had now disappeared (figures and numbers were correctly positioned).

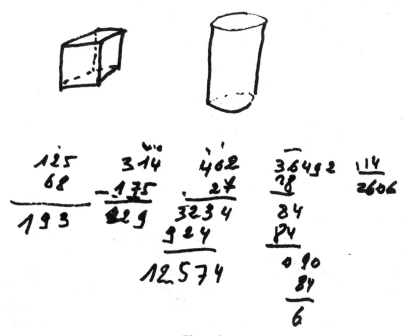

Figure 4

Mathematical abilities were examined independently and rather extensively on two successive days (November 8 and 9) prior to the operation and once again a week after the operation (November 22). Each session lasted for about an hour. The patient was willing to co-operate on all three occasions, even though he complained of tiredness, especially during the first and the third examination.

The purpose of the investigation was to find out in what respect and how severely his mathematical skills were disturbed beyond the execution of basic operations such as addition, subtraction, multiplication and division (these had been tested during the first neuro-linguistic examination on November 6 and it had been found that there was a spatial dyscalculia as well as a genuine anarithmetia. They were, therefore, not re-examined separately, and only appeared within more complex tasks). The investigation consisted of a random succession of problems of the following kind, all of which, unless indicated otherwise, were to be solved in writing:
– completion of simple mathematical series
– labelling of mathematical operations and geometrical figures
– drawing two-dimensional figures
– simplification of algebraic expressions
– formulating the approach to the solution of problems in algebra and geometry
– operations with fractions
– indices and powers
– roots
– interpretation of mathematical symbols
– problems using the metric system
– calculation of the area of geometrical figures
– discovering the axes of symmetrical figures
– simplifying equations with two variables.

Because the patient was a teacher of mathematics he could be expected to have been familiar with such problems.

There was no time limit for the performance of the tasks. A problem was considered 'unsolved' whenever the patient gave up. In case of incorrect answers he was asked whether he was quite sure and given the time to correct himself, which he did in a few instances. He was never told the right answer when he did not find it himself.

Complex problems, such as operations with fractions or the solution of equations generally took him a long time whereas the answers to problems such as squaring, square-roots and labelling of figures were produced rather quickly.

His performance on November 9 did not differ significantly from that on November 8, so that both can be regarded together as the 'pre-operative examination'. A distinct spontaneous improvement

148

was already noticeable by comparison with the neurolinguistic investigation of November 6, because this time multiplications and divisions appearing in other problems could be performed without difficulty.

The post-operative examination, which included most of the operations the patient had not been able to effect pre-operatively, showed an even more considerable improvement. Although it took him more time than might have been expected of a teacher of mathematics, the patient was now capable of solving most of the problems he had had difficulty with before the operation. (The possibility that he might have remembered the correct solution is excluded by the fact that he had not been told it.)

In order to portray as accurately as possible the patient's performance as well as his improvement, it seems best to summarize the results under the following headings:
(1) problems he was able to solve pre-operatively;
(2) problems he was not able to solve pre-operatively;
(3) problems he was not able to solve pre-, but was able to solve post-operatively.

1. *Problems he was able to solve pre-operatively*
The following series, where a certain number had to be added, were continued without difficulties: 2 4 6 ... , $\frac{1}{2}$ 1 $1\frac{1}{2}$ ... , and 1 8 15 22 ... . The correct results were obtained for a number of basic operations with fractions ($\frac{52}{6}$, $\frac{48}{8}$, $\frac{35}{5}$, $\frac{12}{4}$, and $\frac{75}{9}$), one- or two-digit multiplications (3×22, 7×7, 3×9, 9×27, 25×3.14, 30×15, 2×50, 30×60), problems of finding the second or third power of a number (4^2, 3^2, 3^3), and problems of finding the square-root of a number ($\sqrt{25}$, $\sqrt{8}$). The patient labelled correctly examples of addition, subtraction, multiplication and powers, as well as a circle, a triangle, a square, a rectangle, a cube, a pyramid, a cone and a cylinder, and he himself could draw on request a right-angled triangle, a rhombus, a rectangle and a square. He simplified the following algebraic expressions: $a^m \times a^n$, $(a^m)^n$, $(a+b)^2$, $(a+b)(a-b)$, and answered the following questions satisfactorily: How do you calculate the area of a triangle? How do you calculate the volume of a cube? How do you simplify a fraction? What happens if you multiply both terms of a fraction by the same number? How do you multiply the mth power of a number a by the nth power of the same number? How do you

convert a length that is given in metres into centimetres? How much does a litre of water weigh? His knowledge of the mathematical symbols $>$, $<$ and ∞ did not seem to be disturbed as he was able to decide without errors on the correctness or incorrectness of $5>7$, $16<12$, $21\geqslant19$ and $9>7<10$. In addition he knew that the symbol ∞ stands for $\frac{1}{0}$ and not for $\frac{0}{1}$. There were no mistakes in those conversions within the metric system that involved multiplication with small numbers: 1.25 l into cl, 3,500 kg into g, 5,025 dm³ into cm³, 273 cm into mm, 30 min into sec, 30 min into h, nor in the solution of an equation with one variable and four terms: $4x-5=3x+7$. Furthermore, he found the axes for two or more given symmetrical figures, and also correctly calculated the area of a circle with the radius 5 cm and of a rectangle with the sides 30 m and 15 m.

2. Problems he was not able to solve pre-operatively
He continued the series 3 8 5 10 7 12 ..., where addition $(+5)$ and subtraction (-3) had to be alternated, by adding 5 only: 17 22 27 32 37 42. Another alternating series, 55 47 49 41 43 ... $(-8, +2)$ seemed to pose an unsurmountable problem: he could not continue it at all. The same held for the series 27 21 15 ..., where subtraction only is involved. Here again, no solution was offered.

When confronted with the equation $14x-3x-3=5x-10x+27$, he wrote $5x+3x$, which was correct, if he wanted to collect the terms in x on the right side of the equation. He then continued with $+5x+10x$ but realized after a while that there was something wrong, and crossed out the first 5x he had put and added $-$ under $+$ in front of 10x. At this point, he seemed to be completely at a loss about how to proceed. He wrote $+27$ and $=$ and then gave up any further attempt at a solution. He became impatient because he was not able to solve the problem, even though he himself commented that it was rather simple. The next day he had no difficulty with the equation with one variable and four terms mentioned above: $4x-5=3x+7$.

When requested to simplify as far as possible the equation $8a+6-5b-4=9b+5a$, the patient began by rewriting the problem without any changes. He then wrote $+2-5b$ to the left of $=$, and left the right side of the equation unchanged; 8a does not appear at all in this line. The third line consists of $-4=4b+5a$; -4 may have been copied from the first line, even though it seems to have been taken care of in the subtraction $6-4$, the result of which, $+2$, presumably appears in the second line; 4b can only be the result of subtracting 5b from 9b. It should have been added, however.

There were three more complex problems with fractions that could not be solved, at least not at the first attempt:

$$\frac{2-1}{3}+\frac{27+5}{9}$$

was written as

$$\frac{1}{3}+\frac{22}{9}$$

The first term is correct, but the numerator of the second fraction should be 32 instead of 22; 22 may have been the result of subtracting 5 from 27, instead of adding the two numbers. The next line was

$$\frac{9}{9}+\frac{666\!\!\!/}{9};$$

9 in both denominators is correct. Both numerators, however, are incorrect. It appears that he multiplied the numerator of the first fraction by the denominator of the second one and vice-versa, which would have been correct, had the problem been a division between two fractions, instead of an addition. This interpretation is only correct on the assumption that he meant to write 66 instead of 666. (He himself crossed out the last 6 in 6666). This assumption is confirmed by the way he proceeded: his next line is $\frac{75}{9}$, and 75 would be the correct result of the addition between 9 and 66. His solution, $8\frac{1}{3}$, is right with regard to the previous line, but wrong with respect to the original task.

As for $\frac{7}{3}:\frac{9}{7}$, the patient at first wrote $\frac{49}{7}:\frac{27}{}$, that is, he did the required multiplications correctly, but could not write the obtained results in the right position. When asked what you have to do if you want to divide one fraction by another, he was able to formulate verbally what he should have done, and in a second attempt found the correct numerical solution.

When requested to simplify

$$\sqrt{\frac{4x+4}{x+1}},$$

he wrote $\sqrt{8x}$. When asked, whether it is possible to add 4x and 4, the patient quite decidedly said 'no' and crossed out the 'x'. He then proceeded to write $2\sqrt{2}$, which is the correct simplification of $\sqrt{8}$, but not of the original root.

Although he had been able to find lines of symmetry for two or more given symmetrical figures just previously, he found it difficult to detect lines and/or points of symmetry within a given letter. In 'I', for example, he only noticed the point, and neglected the two possible lines of symmetry. He placed a point on the top end of 'A', and drew the line of symmetry only after having been asked whether there should be one or not. For 'S' he gave a perpendicular line without discovering the point, and the line of symmetry in 'W' was not detected at all.

He converted 25 min to 15000$\emptyset$ sec (he himself crossed out the last zero), 273 cm to 0.25 m, and 5,260 kg to 42,600,000 g. For the conversions of 25 min to hours, 273 cm to km and 5,260 g to mg, no solution was offered at all.

When asked to calculate the area of a rectangle, the sides of which were given as 2 m and 50 cm, he wrote 'S$=$100'. His attention was drawn to the fact that the sides were given in different units. It took him quite a time to grasp what was wrong with his solution. In the end he wrote $50 \times 200\emptyset$, multiplied the numbers correctly, but converted 10,000 cm^2 into 10, again without unit.

3. *Problems he was not able to solve pre-, but was able to solve post-operatively*

During the examination which took place after the operation, the patient was asked to do again some of these problems he had had difficulty with, or had not been able to solve pre-operatively. This time he produced the right answers easily and without apparent effort. He correctly continued the series involving subtraction only (27 21 15 ...), and one of the series alternating between subtraction and addition: 55 47 49 41 43 .... He calculated the area of the rectangle mentioned above (with the side-lengths 2 m and 50 cm), simplified

$$\sqrt{\frac{4x+4}{x+1}} \text{ to } 2$$

and solved the equation $14x-3x-3=5x-10x+27$. In addition, he simplified

$$\frac{\sqrt{(a-b)^2}}{a-b}+\frac{1}{\sqrt{\frac{16-12}{25}}},$$

drew several three-dimensional figures correctly, and found the graphical representations of the functions $y=x^2$, $y=2x+1$, and $y=x^3$.

Discussion

In order to find out the exact nature of our patient's dyscalculia, it seems best to begin with an analysis of the difficulties he had, or the type of errors he made.

A possible way to approach the recognition of a mathematical series is to compare any two numbers (generally the first pair), infer from these a hypothesis, and then check this hypothesis with the help of the rest of the sequence. Should this hypothesis prove to be wrong, another one will have to be formulated, checked, and so on, until the conjecture finally matches the series. The patient was able to continue correctly 2 4 6 ..., $\frac{1}{2}$ 1 $1\frac{1}{2}$ ..., and 1 8 15 22 ..., but not 3 8 5 10 7 12 ..., 55 47 49 41 43 ..., and 27 21 15 .... The possibility that his ability to do subtractions was impaired is excluded by the fact that he subtracted correctly in other instances. It rather seems to be the case that his difficulty lay in giving up the first hypothesis that came to his mind and formulating a new one, when the first proved false. His first hypothesis was probably that the series had to be continued by addition. This can be inferred from the first pair of numbers in all but the last two series, and is only incorrect for the fourth one, which he nevertheless continued by addition. The last two examples, which start with subtraction, were not continued at all. He might have noticed that his first hypothesis was incorrect, without being able to think of another one. Something rather similar can be said about the tasks of finding lines and/or points of symmetry for symmetrical figures or for symmetrical letters. Here one has to form a hypothesis by imagining a certain line or point, check whether it is an axis, accept this hypothesis if it is correct, abandon it and formulate a new one if it proves to be wrong. Again, the patient was able to do this when the first hypothesis that presumably came to his mind happened to be correct, as in the detection of axes for symmetrical figures. As soon as the task became somewhat more intricate, that is, as soon as there were several acceptable solutions, he began making mistakes, presumably because he was unable to abandon the first possibility he had thought of, as in 'A' and 'S'. For 'I' the first solution was correct, but he could not go on to find the other one.

In one case ('W') he was unable to propose any solution at all. Possibly, again, he noticed that his first hypothesis was incorrect but could not think of another one.

As regards the solution of an equation with one variable, one should realize that what one is required to do is to figure out the value of x. Thus, the task is to collect terms in x on one side of the equation sign, those without x on the other side, add or subtract as is appropriate, and finally divide the whole equation by the remaining factor of x. The patient was able to follow this procedure in the simple case $4x-5=3x+7$, where not even the final division is required, but in the more complicated problem $14x-3x-3=5x-10x+27$, there seemed to be a confusion between the collection of terms in x and those without x on the right side. In the simplification of $8a+6-5b-4=9b+5a$ he ignored the subtraction $6-4$ carried out just previously. His subtraction of 5b from 9b when he ought to have added them could either be explained by a confusion of the two processes or by perseveration, since the preceding operation was also a subtraction. The fact that neither 14x nor 8a, the two left-most terms, appeared in the solution could be explained by a neglect in the left field of vision. Both equations were abandoned because of his inability to go on.

In the problem

$$\frac{2-1}{3}+\frac{27+5}{9}$$

we first find a confusion between addition and subtraction ($27-5$ instead of $27+5$), which again, could be due to perseveration; 6666 seems to be a clear example of unnecessary reduplication. In what follows the patient chose operations that were appropriate for the division between two fractions instead of performing the actions necessary for finding the common denominator and thus being able to add them. These two somewhat complex processes were, in reversed order, mixed up in the solution of $\frac{7}{3}:\frac{9}{7}$. Writing the results of the multiplications in the numerators would have been correct had the problem required an addition instead of a division between two fractions.

For the proposed simplification of

$$\sqrt{\frac{4x+4}{x+1}}$$

it could be that the patient simply was not aware of the fact that there was a fraction within the square-root. On the assumption that he only noticed the numerator, one can speculate that he confused the processes of adding and multiplying two terms with different variables: the latter can be done but not the former, which he tried to do nevertheless.

The mistakes in those conversions within the metric system which he performed incorrectly seem to be due to reduplication (15,000 instead of 1,500), possibly complicated by some visual field defect (42,600,000 instead of 5,260,000). In the other cases there is an inability to propose a solution at all, but for a different reason. To be able to convert within the metric system, one has to compare the two units involved, realize how often one is contained in the other, and multiply or divide the number by this factor, as appropriate. This can be done almost automatically with common conversions such as kg into g or m into cm, but when the task is more complex, one has to become consciously aware of the strategy. When comparing the problems our patient solved (correctly or incorrectly) with those he was not able to solve at all, it seems that he could perform the more automatic conversions, but failed in the less automatic ones. Good examples are the expression of 30 min respectively 25 min in terms of hours: in each case the process involved is division by 60 because there are 60 minutes in an hour. But while the former conversion is rather common and was performed without effort, the latter one requires a realization of the necessary steps involved, and this he was not able to do.

In the calculation of the area of the rectangle 2 m × 50 cm, he immediately started multiplying without realizing that he had to convert the units first. So the error he made here consists in the omission of the conversion.

In summary several types of errors were produced during the examination:

(a) errors which are visuo-spatial in nature such as reduplication of figures and occasional neglect of left-most numbers, for instance in equations;

(b) errors which appear to be due to some inertia or a tendency to repeat the same pattern of behaviour instead of shifting to a new one, such as his inability to abandon a hypothesis and formulate a new one in the continuation of a series, or the performance of two subtractions in succession, where the second operation should have been an addition;

(c) errors which consist of the omission of a necessary step or the mixing up of several stages of a somewhat complex operation, the confusion perhaps being partly due to perseveration or to visual field defects;

(d) genuine arithmetic mistakes. These were of two sorts. In some cases, the patient erred because he mixed up two different strategies, as when he applied parts of the techniques for dividing fractions to what should have been an addition of fractions, or when he confused the processes of adding and multiplying two terms with different variables. In some other cases he could offer no solution at all. When considering these arithmetic mistakes it appears that our patient did not stumble over one particular type of operation (as in the cases reported by Berger, 1926). Rather, his difficulties resulted from the complexity of the operation. This can be clearly seen if one compares the problems he was able to solve with those he could not solve: He continued $2\ 4\ 6\ ...$ but not $3\ 8\ 5\ 10\ 7\ 12\ ...$; he solved $4x-5=3x+7$ but not $14x-3x-3=5x-10x+27$; he calculated the area of the rectangle $30\ m \times 15\ m$ but not of $2\ m \times 50\ cm$; he converted 30 min into hours but not 25 min, and so forth. All of the more complex problems require an awareness of the goal to be achieved, and a realization of the steps that are necessary to achieve it – that is, the development of some strategy. The patient was either unable to conceive a strategy or to retain a strategy once it had been started.

It is not surprising to find the errors listed under (a): reduplications and unilateral neglect could also be observed in the writing of sentences, as the neurolinguistic examination revealed. Such errors are typical of the visuo-spatial dyscalculia which has been described in dextrals with right brain damage.

The second type of errors made by our patient was due to perseveration or inertia. A tendency to perseverate has been found in the metalinguistic behaviour of patients with right frontal lesions (Marcie *et al.*, 1965), and in the performance of mathematical operations by patients with right frontal damage (Luria and Tsvetkova, 1967).

Errors similar to those mentioned under (c) have also been described by Benson and Weir (1972). They found that 'only during multidigit multiplication did the patient err. A number of steps are carried out simultaneously during this process – these include retrieval of the multiplication tables, appropriate spatial alignment of the digits and retention and appropriate use of any integers remaining from the previous product (carrying). These steps are performed almost simultaneously, essentially as a single step, by most educated individuals. Our patient could not introspectively separate the steps to discover where his prime difficulty lay. Similarly, observations by the examiners failed to isolate any single step as the source of the failure. Nonetheless, it would appear that a confusion of the processes (adding, multiplying and carrying) was the source of his consistent calculation disturbance.' (p. 471)

Interestingly enough, Benson and Weir's patient had a lesion in the dominant hemisphere while our patient had suffered right brain damage.

The errors listed under (d) are probably the most interesting ones. Neither visual field defect nor perseveration or inertia can account for them, and they appear to be genuine arithmetic mistakes. The mixing up of different strategies is not rare in patients with a left-sided lesion. Lindqvist (1935), for instance, observed the execution of addition instead of subtraction and of addition instead of multiplication in a patient with left brain damage. Similar confusions were also present in a (presumably) bilateral case of carbon monoxide poisoning described by Singer and Low (1933). Here multiplication instead of addition, addition instead of multiplication, and subtraction instead of addition were performed. However, Bresson et al. (1972) insist that this kind of error is more frequent in connection with right-sided lesions. Similar confusions, although they are not mentioned explicitly, seem also to have been present in the performance of the patients with right frontal lesions whom Luria and Tsvetkova (1967) described.

Again, in his inability to conceive or retain a strategy in complex operations, our patient fits almost exactly the description given by Luria and Tsvetkova (1967) of disturbances of the intellectual abilities due to lesions of the frontal lobes: 'En règle générale, l'exécution d'opérations bien acquises reste dans ces cas relativement bien conservée. (...) Ces malades n'analysent pas les données du problème qui leur est posé, (...) Ils n'établissent pas de schéma ou de programme général de résolution du problème à partir de l'analyse préliminaire de ses données, et se limitent le plus souvent à essayer de donner des réponses impulsives à certains éléments des données qui, on ne sait pourquoi, ont pu retenir leur attention et ont été dégagées de l'ensemble.' (p. 9–10).

This case of dyscalculia in a right-handed teacher of mathematics thus shows that a lesion of the minor hemisphere may cause not only visuo-spatial computation disorders but also genuine anarithmetia. In our patient, the anarithmetia comprised calculating errors, occasional confusion of the fundamental operations, and a difficulty to take simultaneously into account the various components of a problem and to keep apart the various stages of a resolution. Moreover, the patient sometimes failed to remember the methods through which some typical mathematical task could be performed. This anarithmetia was complicated by a tendency to perseveration.

7

LANGUAGE FUNCTIONS IN HEMISPHERECTOMIZED PATIENTS

YVAN LEBRUN, CHANTAL LELEUX

In 1973 the Norwegian neuroanatomist A. Brodal published a paper in which he learnedly described the sequelae of a stroke he had sustained a few months earlier. Dysarthria, disturbances of handwriting and comprehension difficulties were among the symptoms he mentioned.

Brodal's dysarthria was incommensurate with his central facial paresis and receded more slowly than the motor deficit. Six months after the stroke, it was still present and tended to increase when the patient was tired.

Writing disturbances included uneven and oblique lines, duplications and omissions of strokes and letters and occasionally of words, figure inversions, irregularly shaped letters and spacing of letters within words.

Although by clinical and even psychometrical standards he was not aphasic (on the WAIS he scored a verbal IQ of 142), Brodal felt that he had difficulty following the line of argument in scientific papers. Subjectively this difficulty seemed to result from 'a reduction of short-term memory for abstract symbols'.

Thus, although he was right-handed and his left hemisphere in all likelihood had sustained no damage, Brodal was left with a moderate verbal impairment after a stroke in the right hemisphere. Quite logically the author concluded that for optimal linguistic functioning, we need a whole brain. This implies that even in dextrals, the so-called minor hemisphere is not without significance for verbal processes and that a lesion of this hemisphere 'while producing no clinically apparent aphasia, may nonetheless give rise to subtle defects in the linguistic sphere,' to quote Zangwill's words (1967).

As a matter of fact, Penfield and his co-workers have observed that

159

vocalization or arrest of speech may result from electrical stimulation of motor areas on the non-dominant side (Penfield and Roberts, 1959, pp. 121 and 131). According to Eisenson (1962), right-handed patients with right brain damage perform less proficiently on vocabulary selection tests and sentence completion tests than matched control subjects without cerebral lesion. Marcie and colleagues (1965) have observed that dextrals with right hemispheric damage tend to repeat nonsense words less accurately than normal subjects; in addition, some of these patients have difficulty forming a sentence which contains words given by the examiner. This latter finding has been confirmed by Assal and Zander (1969). There are indications that right brain damaged patients find it difficult to answer correctly such questions as *John is taller than Bill, who is shorter?* (Caramazza *et al.*, 1976). It has also been noticed that damage to the non-dominant hemisphere may render the patient abnormally verbose and prone to digression (Lebrun, 1974). A lesion in the non-dominant half of the brain may easily entail an afferent dysgraphia (Lebrun, 1976) and reading difficulties (Lebrun, 1974). It has been observed that a right hemispheric lesion may significantly impair the comprehension of affective speech, i.e. the identification of moods (such as happiness or indifference) expressed by the pitch or tone of the voice (Heilman *et al.*, 1975). Right brain damaged patients tend to have more difficulty identifying voices than left brain damaged patients and normals (Assal, Buttet and Zander, this volume). These various findings are consonant with the observation made in Copenhagen (Larsen *et al.*, 1978; Lassen *et al.*, 1978) that verbal activities increase the regional blood flow in similar regions of *both* hemispheres.

It thus appears that while the two cerebral hemispheres are certainly not equipotential as regards verbal skills, nonetheless both of them are involved in language processing, so that even a lesion in the minor hemisphere may disturb at least some aspects of the use of language. It is therefore all the more striking when extensive damage to the supposedly dominant hemisphere fails to entail any noteworthy deficit, as in the case described below.

Up to November 1977, the patient had been well. She was from right-handed stock and was herself right-handed. She was 45 years old and worked as a fashion stylist. On November 6 she had an epileptic fit during which she lost consciousness. She was admitted to the neurosurgical department (Prof. Dr. J. Brihaye) for examination.

160

The EEG showed anomalies over the left temporal area while both brain scan and arteriogram pointed to a vast tumor occupying most of the temporal lobe and invading part of the frontal and parietal lobes. Clinical neurological examination was normal, except for an exaggerated rotulian reflex on the right. Neuropsychological investigation revealed an impairment of verbal short-term memory and a difficulty recalling proper nouns.

On November 10, 1977, a craniotomy was performed. The tumor appeared to be large and primarily subcortical. Only a small part of it was excised, which proved to be of an infiltrating astrocytoma.

Post-operatively, the patient was given a thorough neurolinguistic examination.

Simple and semi-complex orders were executed promptly and correctly. Complex orders (e.g. Marie's three-paper-test) could be understood but not remembered long enough to allow faultless execution. Pointing to objects or to body parts named by the examiner caused no difficulty whatsoever. There was no right–left confusion.

Spontaneous speech was fluent, copious and errorless.

Familiar objects could easily be named. Subtle shades of colour could be distinguished verbally (e.g. turquoise blue, claret wine, bottle green ...).

However, the patient complained that she could not remember the date and had great difficulty committing new proper nouns to memory. As a matter of fact, during her stay in the hospital she could never remember the names of the physicians who were in charge of the ward. On the other hand, names of relatives and of friends she had known for a long time could be easily recalled.

The patient could produce series of words belonging to a given semantic field (e.g. names of animals, of flowers, of musical instruments). She could turn masculine forms into feminine, give antonyms and produce rhyming or alliterating words.

Written commands were executed correctly, even complex ones.

Spontaneous writing and writing under dictation evidenced no anomaly and her handwriting was neat and legible (see Fig. 1). Spelling words aloud from memory was errorless.

Reading aloud was correct. However, when the patient had to retell a story she had just been reading, she omitted a number of features. She spontaneously commented that when she was reading a

Je suis en traitement dans l'hôpital. Je subis les traitements nécessaires en espérant qu'ils seront tous salutaires et efficaces.

A certains endroits le vint a soufflé à plus de 100 kms heure

La neige a commencé à tomber dans les Ardennes

La tempête a commis de gros dégats surtout en Belgique

En mer et en Angleterre elle a été meurtrière

J'étais dessinatrice de mode.

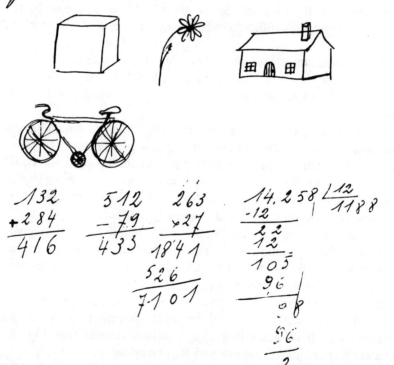

Figure 1

book she frequently had to go back a few pages, for she had forgotten what she had just been reading.

There was a slight mental dyscalculia, but the patient insisted that she had never been able to calculate mentally without errors. Her written arithmetic was correct (Figure 1).

She could draw very well, as Figures 2 and 3 show.

She was not disoriented and could locate the main Belgian towns on a blank map of Belgium.

Conventional gesture language was undisturbed. Transitive as well as intransitive movements were executed promptly and correctly on request and the imitation of meaningless gestures was perfect.

There was no finger agnosia, no colour agnosia, no prosopagnosia (but the patient could not always remember the name of the celebrity shown), no astereognosia. There was perhaps a slight impairment of dermolexia (or hypoesthesia) on the right side.

There was no avocalia.

In short, apart from a difficulty remembering new proper nouns and retaining new verbal material, the neurolinguistic examination did not reveal the slightest anomaly.

The absence of neurological symptoms and the very small number of neurolinguistic shortcomings are very striking in view of the localization and the extent of the lesion. To be sure, the tumor appeared to be primarily subcortical and there is no postmortem verification of it. Nonetheless, on the basis of the CAT scan, which evidenced a large hypodense zone in the temporal lobe (Fig. 4) and of the arteriogram, which indicated that the sylvian artery was displaced upwards and to the right, one might have expected rather severe aphasic disturbances in the patient.

How comes that her impairment was so restricted?

A first explanation would be that she belonged to the small group of dextrals whose right hemisphere is dominant for language. If this was the case, then it should be emphasized that her cortical organization was not simply a mirror-image of what is commonly found in dextrals: her left hemisphere did not seem to fulfil the functions which are usually those of the non-dominant hemisphere in right-handed people. None of the difficulties mentioned at the beginning of this paper was observed. In particular, the disorders of writing and drawing, which are so frequently found in dextrals whose right hemisphere has been damaged, did not obtain in this case.

163

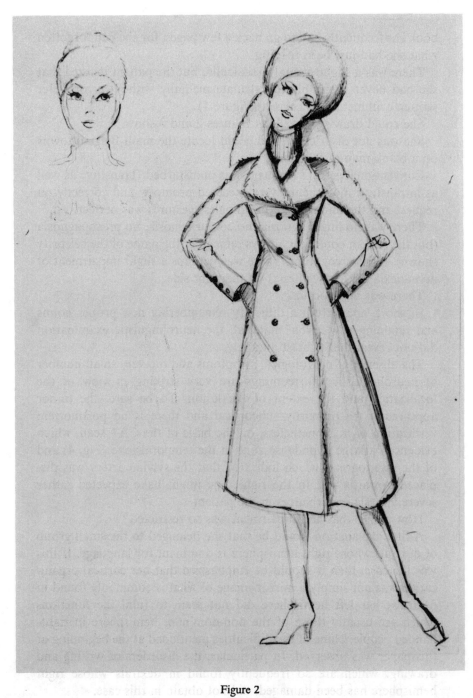

Figure 2

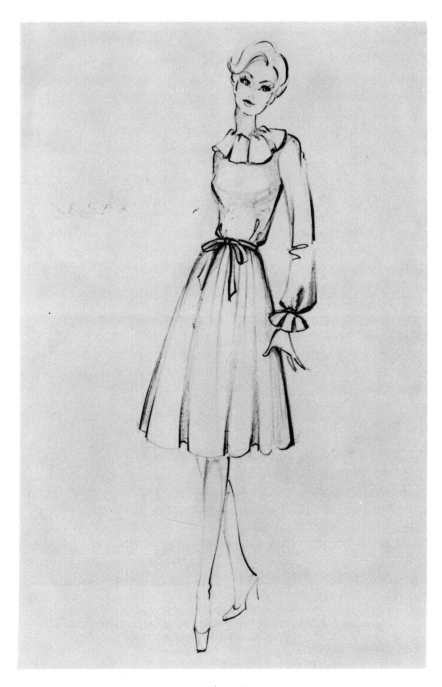

Figure 3

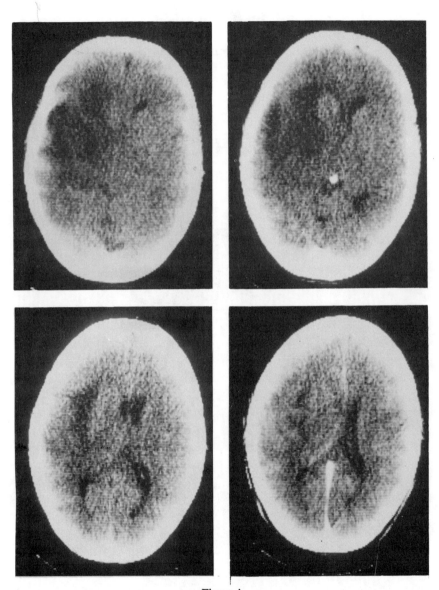

Figure 4

(By courtesy of D. Balériaux-Waha, M.D., Service de radiodiagnostic,
Institut Jules Bordet, Brussels)

Another possibility is that her left hemisphere was originally
dominant for language, but, as her tumor grew slowly, the patient

166

was able to compensate for the damage it was causing. Some thirty years ago, Walther Riese (1949) pointed out that slowly growing neoplasms may develop in speech areas without entailing aphasia: 'The organism can maintain undisturbed functions for a long time in spite of massive lesions destroying or damaging the critical areas of these functions, provided the lesions have a slow momentum.'* Riese further suggested that the unimpaired functions are taken over by spared tissue. In the case reported above, it is not possible to know whether linguistic functions were transferred to intact parts within the dominant hemisphere or, on the contrary, to homologous parts of the other hemisphere. One might be tempted to reason that if the linguistic functions had been taken over by the minor hemisphere, the verbal competence of the patient should have been rather limited, as one hemisphere alone can hardly be supposed to achieve as much as two hemispheres together. The validity of such reasoning can be tested, it would seem, by examining the linguistic proficiency of individuals who have undergone hemidecortication or hemispherectomy. In these patients, language functions are necessarily dependent on only one hemisphere. What are the verbal performances of such persons? Can one hemisphere achieve as much linguistic proficiency as a complete telencephalon? And is there a difference between the capacities of the isolated left hemisphere and those of the isolated right hemisphere?

Some authorities seem to be of the opinion that the prospects of reaching normal verbal competence are good when the lesion that has rendered hemispherectomy necessary was incurred early in life. Gazzaniga and Hillyard (1971), for instance, state that 'the right hemisphere is potentially capable of almost normal language and speech function' and in case of hemispherectomy can assume these duties with little or no difficulty if the insulting events to the left hemisphere occur at an early age. Zangwill (1967) seems to entertain a similar view: 'Speech may develop normally following severe left hemisphere damage at birth or in early infancy and later removal of the damaged hemisphere (hemispherectomy) does not as a rule give rise to aphasia.' Lhermitte (1968) is even more positive: 'L'ablation de tout un hémisphère – le droit ou le gauche – chez l'enfant n'ayant

---

* As a matter of fact, as early as 1836, Marc Dax alluded to the possibility that a slowly developing disease of the left hemisphere might entail no language disorder (Dax, 1865).

pas dépassé 12 ans, ne détermine pas l'apparition de troubles du langage, sinon d'une manière tout éphémère.'

Such statements imply that it is possible to develop normal or quasi-normal verbal skills with only one hemisphere, provided the hemispherectomy is performed early in life. Moreover, it does not matter whether the left or the right hemisphere is removed.

Not everybody shares this optimistic view. Some authors doubt whether hemispherectomized individuals can achieve normal command of language when the remaining hemisphere was originally non-dominant. 'We are all appreciative of the alleged plasticity of the infant brain,' Teuber stated at a conference held at Princeton in 1965, 'but we do not seem to have any strong evidence to suggest that the lateralization of different functions can really be reversed with complete impunity.' According to Teuber, the risk of having 'diminished ultimate language competence' is considerable when the dominant hemisphere is removed in a child (see Millikan and Darley, 1967, p. 213).

In view of these conflicting opinions, it seems worthwhile to examine the available clinical and experimental data regarding linguistic skills in hemispherectomized subjects.

In trying to ascertain the effects of hemispherectomy on language, it is desirable to distinguish patients who undergo hemispherectomy at an early age, mostly in order to relieve symptoms of infantile hemiplegia, from adults who are hemispherectomized because of cerebral neoplasm.

One is generally agreed that left hemispherectomy in right-handed adults brings about a very severe and long-lasting aphasia. In the few patients who have survived the operation for some appreciable length of time, limited language recovery could be observed. In a case described by Smith (1966) partly in collaboration with Burklund (1966), comprehension of simple speech was present shortly after operation. Understanding of spoken language increased with time. Eventually, auditory comprehension as judged clinically reached a near normal level (Smith, 1972). Immediately after operation, the patient was heard to use expletives but he had no propositional speech. With time, however, he regained the ability to occasionally use short propositional sentences. He also made some limited progress in reading and writing.

Right-sided hemispherectomy in right-handed adults affects language

168

far less than removal of the left side of the brain. As an example the case reported by Gott (1973) may be quoted. The patient was a thirty-four year old right-handed female, whose formal education included three years at college level. When she was twenty-eight the patient was operated upon because of cerebral neoplasm and her right hemisphere was removed but for the basal ganglia. Test results indicated that language was essentially normal. However, Gott's battery did not tap any of the rather subtle linguistic skills which are usually found to be disturbed in dextrals with right brain damage, as was indicated as the beginning of this paper. It is therefore possible that the right hemispherectomy which Gott's patient underwent, did not leave her linguistic competence fully intact. It is also possible that the patient evidenced some verbal deficits after hemispherectomy but learned to compensate for them in the six years' period between operation and testing. A third alternative is that the chronogenesis of her cerebral tumor was slow, so that the verbal duties generally fulfilled by the right hemisphere could be progressively taken over by the other side of the brain. A similar transfer, but in opposite direction, may have taken place in the fashion stylist described above.

Interestingly enough, Gott's patient found acquisition of new knowledge difficult, mainly because of an impairment of short-term memory. Although Gott does not indicate whether this included *verbal* short-term memory, it may be presumed that it did, since such a defect, as was mentioned above, was subjectively felt to be present in Brodal (1973), and could be shown to exist in the right brain damaged dextral described by Leleux, Kaiser and Lebrun in this volume (p. 145). Accordingly, Gott's conclusion that 'two hemispheres appear to be necessary, or at least greatly facilitatory, in the acquisition of new knowledge' in all likelihood also applies to language. This in turn explains why the only neuropsychological impairment which could be detected in the fashion stylist described in this paper was precisely a difficulty retaining new verbal material.

Ablation of one cerebral hemisphere at a younger age does not appear to be so detrimental to the acquisition of new knowledge, including verbal knowledge. Smith and Sugar (1975) have reported the case of an industrial executive who had undergone left hemispherectomy when he was 5.5 years old. Intractable rightsided Jacksonian seizures had motivated the operation, which spared only the left basal ganglia and some ependyma of the left temporal horn.

Some fifteen years after surgery this patient had a Wechsler verbal IQ of 113 and a Peabody Picture Vocabulary Test score of 125. Six years later, the former score had increased by 13, while the latter was above 137. Clinically, his speech, language comprehension, reading and writing appeared to be normal. Accordingly, Smith and Sugar concluded that 'following removal of the left hemisphere, including "the classical zones of language", the right hemisphere and other residual structures may provide the necessary substrata for the development of above normal language.' While this may be true, it should be remembered that the test battery used by Smith and Sugar tapped but a limited number of linguistic capacities. After all, Brodal (1973) had no language deficit by clinical standards and he had a Wechsler verbal IQ of 142. He nonetheless felt that he had suffered some verbal loss, some reduction of his verbal abilities.

Whether or not an extensive test battery might have uncovered some less developed linguistic capabilities, it is clear that with only one hemisphere Smith and Sugar's patient managed to acquire the verbal skills which his position as an industrial executive required.

Interestingly enough, this patient significantly improved his verbal score between age 20 and age 26: it looks as if his language development though it had not been limited by the removal of the left hemisphere, yet took place at a slower pace. Some support for this hypothesis derives from a study by Dennis and Whitaker (1977), who administered the Illinois Test of Psycholinguistic Abilities to three 9 year 5 month old children: two of them had undergone early left hemispherectomy and the third one early right hemispherectomy because of intractable seizures that were part of their Sturge-Weber-Dimitri syndrome. Their composite psycholinguistic ages proved to be very similar: 7.9, 7.3, and 7.8 respectively. Thus the three children showed some two years' delay in language development.

Although the scores on the various subtests indicated large inter- and intra-individual variability, the overall verbal score of the right hemidecorticate was not superior to the overall scores of the left hemidecorticates. This observation is consonant with the findings of McFie (1961), who gave the Wechsler-Bellevue test battery to two children who had undergone left hemispherectomy and four who had undergone right hemispherectomy. The highest verbal score (97) was reached by a subject whose left hemisphere had been removed and the lowest by a subject whose right hemisphere had been resected. In

170

addition, the two left hemidecorticates and three of the four right hemidecorticates were given Weigl's sorting test before and after operation. Pre-operatively, none of the children was able to pass the test. Post-operatively, the two left hemidecorticates and only one of the three right hemidecorticates could pass it. Thus, as regards language development, children who undergo early right hemispherectomy are not necessarily better off than children who undergo early left hemispherectomy. Indeed, Smith and Sugar's case shows that the right hemisphere can achieve good command of language by itself.

To be sure, Dennis and Kohn (1975), comparing the syntactical comprehension of right and left hemidecorticates matched for overall verbal IQ, found the right hemidecorticates to be superior for comprehension of passive sentences (there was no difference between the two groups as regards understanding of active sentences). Dennis and Kohn concluded, accordingly, that 'a more extended language development is possible in a remaining left hemisphere.' It should be pointed out, however, that their left hemispherectomy subjects were operated upon at the age of 10 years 6 months, 14 years 6 months, 13 years 11 months, 17 years 10 months, and 5 months, respectively. But for one, these subjects were adolescents or even young adults when they were hemispherectomized. It may therefore be wondered whether the test scores of such hemidecorticates should not be interpreted in terms of language loss rather than in terms of language development. Moreover, the one subject who underwent early hemispherectomy and who was tested when he was 8 years old understood correctly all the active affirmative sentences and 90% of the active negative sentences but reached chance level in the interpretation of passive sentences. This seems to be more typical of a slow than of a restricted language development. It would appear, therefore, that if there is really a difference in language acquisition between left and right hemispherectomy individuals, this difference may relate more to the speed than to the extent of acquisition.

At any rate, the attainment of linguistic proficiency with half a brain appears to be rare. Only one of the nine hemispherectomees examined by Dennis and Kohn understood virtually all the test sentences. Still, seven of them were adults at the time of testing. Most probably, the acquisition of adequate verbal functions necessitates at least one intact hemisphere, and in many individuals who undergo early hemispherectomy the remaining hemisphere may not be quite healthy.

Nonetheless, removal of one side of the brain does increase verbal competence in a number of children with infantile cerebral injuries. Each of the six hemispherectomees examined by McFie (1961) improved his verbal IQ by several points after operation. And Heuyer and Feld (1954) have reported the case of a boy who following encephalitis at eleven months started to have severe seizures. Five months later, he developed a right-sided hemiplegia. Behavioural disorders soon appeared, while the child failed to acquire language. When the patient was three and a half, the left hemisphere, which appeared to be atrophied, was resected. Following operation, the hemiplegia became less severe, the disorders of behaviour decreased and linguistic functions started to develop. A year and a half later, the boy could freely converse with his relatives.

Indeed, hemispherectomy can be beneficial to language even when it is performed in adulthood. Griffith and Davidson (1966) have described a patient who started having seizures at the age of ten and hemiplegia at twelve. A right hemispherectomy was performed at the age of nineteen. Before operation, the patient's verbal IQ was 101. One year after operation, it was 119 and some fifteen years later 121. Moreover, the patient appeared post-operatively to be less verbose and less digressive.

In this case it would seem that the right hemisphere, although it was diseased, yet attempted to play its part in language processing: pre-operatively the patient presented a symptom which can be observed in a number of dextrals with right brain damage, namely verbosity and digressiveness (see above). Hemispherectomy probably put an end to the inadequate contribution of the right side of the brain to linguistic activity: the patient's speech became terser and his verbal IQ improved after operation.

A similar situation may have obtained in the case reported by Heuyer and Feld. The left hemisphere through direct though inappropriate participation in verbal processes may have impeded rather than furthered language development. An alternative possibility is that the left hemisphere was too atrophied to take part in language acquisition but through the seizures it caused prevented the other half of the brain from developing any verbal skills. As a matter of fact, the disruptions provoked by the damaged hemisphere may

172

be so severe as to render the patient virtually oligophrenic. Damasio *et al.* (1975) have described a woman who had been healthy until she was five years old, when she sustained a severe closed head injury. When she was examined at the age of eight she had a marked left hemiplegia. Four years later, she began to have left-sided focal seizures. On examination at the age of eighteen she was found to have aggressive and disturbed behaviour and was considered oligophrenic. Her diseased right hemisphere was removed two years later after grand mal seizures had become frequent and uncontrollable. The EEG before operation showed a poor alpha rhythm with diffuse slow waves on both hemispheres and spike and wave activity in the right frontal leads. After the hemispherectomy, the fits subsided completely without further medication and serial EEGs of the left side of the brain proved to be normal. Fourteen years after surgery the patient's command of oral and written language was found to be adequate and her behaviour was unremarkable.

It thus appears that it is not impossible to achieve linguistic proficiency with only one cerebral hemisphere, whether it is the left or the right hemisphere that was damaged in early youth and has had to be removed. However, not many hemidecorticates have been reported to have attained adequate command of language, probably because in the majority of patients with infantile cerebral lesions who undergo hemispherectomy, the remaining brain half is not intact. Moreover, even when the left-over hemisphere is healthy, language development seems to be slower, at least in left hemispherectomy subjects.* Nonetheless, in a number of cases removal of one cerebral hemisphere proves to be beneficial to language development, as the hemisphere injured in early life may prevent the patient from developing any linguistic skills or may cause verbal dysfunctions which resemble those observed in adults with acquired disorders of language.

* This may explain why the right hemidecorticate to whom Dennis and Whitaker (1976) administered various verbal tests when he was nine and a half, ten and a half, and almost eleven years old, was found to be in *some* respects superior to two left hemidecorticates who were given the same tests when they were eight, nine, and nine and a half years old.

173

REFERENCES

AJAX, E. (1967) *Dyslexia without agraphia*. Neurology 17: 645–652.
AJAX E., SCHENKENBERG T., KOSTELJANETZ M. (1977) *Alexia without agraphia and the inferior splenium*. Neurology 27: 685–688.
AJURIAGUERRA J. (1965) *Sprachstörungen beim Kind und Hemisphärendominanz*. Wiener Zeitschrift für Nervenheilkunde und deren Grenzgebiete 22: 1–27.
AJURIAGUERRA J., HECAEN H. (1960) *Le cortex cérébral*. Paris, Masson.
AJURIAGUERRA J., TISSOT R. (1969) *The apraxias*. In VINKEN P., BRUYN G. (eds.) *Handbook of clinical neurology* 4. Amsterdam, North-Holland Publishing Company: 48–66.
ALAJOUANINE T. (1968) *L'aphasie et le langage pathologique*. Paris, Baillière.
ALAJOUANINE T., LHERMITTE F. (1964) *Nonverbal communication in aphasia*. In DEREUCK A. V. S., O'CONNOR M. (eds.) *Disorders of language*. Boston, Little, Brown, and Company: 168–182.
ALAJOUANINE T., LHERMITTE F. (1965) *Acquired aphasia in children*. Brain 88: 653–662.
ALAJOUANINE T., LHERMITTE F., LEDOUX M., RENAUD D., and VIGNOLO L. A. (1964) *Les composantes phonémiques et sémantiques de la jargonaphasie*. Revue Neurologique 110: 5–20.
ALAJOUANINE T., SABOURAUD O. and RIBAUCOURT B. DE (1952) *Désintégration anosognosique des valeurs sémantiques du langage*. Journal de Psychologie 45: 158–180/293–330.
ALBERT M., SPARKS R., HELM N. (1973) *Melodic intonation therapy for aphasia*. Archives of Neurology 22: 130–131.
ANASTASOPOULOS G., KOKKINI D. (1962) *Cerebral dominance and localisation of the language functions*. Psychiatria et Neurologia 143: 6–19.
ARISTOTE (1969). *De l'interprétation*. Edition TRICOT (Paris), Vrin.
ASSAL G. (1965) *Au sujet de l'aphasie et du problème des localisations cérébrales*. Revue Médicale de la Suisse Romande 85: 559–571.
ASSAL G. (1973) *Aphasie de Wernicke sans amusie chez un pianiste*. Revue Neurologique 129: 251–255.
ASSAL G., BUTTET J., JAVET R. (1977) *Aptitudes musicales chez les aphasiques*. Revue Médicale de la Suisse Romande 97: 5–12.
ASSAL G., GAILLARD G. (1972). *A propos de la reconnaissance auditive chez*

175

l'aphasique: le problème de la discrimination des intonations. Communication at the Schweizerische Arbeitsgemeinschaft für Logopädie (SAL), Zürich.

ASSAL G., ZANDER E. (1969) *Rappel de la symptomatologie neuropsychologique des lésions hémisphériques droites*. Archives Suisses de Neurologie, Neurochirurgie et Psychiatrie 105: 217–239.

ASSAL G., ZANDER E. (1975) *Anomie et alexie lors d'un traumatisme cranio-cérébral fermé*. Neuro-Chirurgie 21: 591–596.

ASSAL G., ZANDER E., KREMIN H, BUTTET J. (1976) *Discrimination des voix lors des lésions du cortex cérébral*. Archives Suisses de Neurologie, de Neurochirurgie et de Psychiatrie, 119: 307–315.

BARTHOLOMEUS B. (1974) *Effects of task requirements on ear superiority for sung speech*. Cortex 10: 215–223.

BARUK H., BERTRAND I., HARTMANN E. (1928) *Un cas d'alexie traumatique*. Revue Neurologique: 287–292.

BASSO A., DE RENZI P., FAGLIONI P., SCOTTI G., SPINNLER H. (1973) *Neuropsychological evidence for the existence of cerebral areas critical to the performance of intelligence tasks*. Brain 96: 715–728.

BAY E. (1949) *Über die sogenannte motorische Aphasie*. Der Nervenarzt 20: 481–490.

BAY E. (1957) *Die corticale Dysarthrie und ihre Beziehung zur sogenannten motorischen Aphasie*. Deutsche Zeitschrift für Nervenheilkunde 176: 553–495.

BAY E. (1960) *Zur Methodik der Aphasie-Untersuchung*. Der Nervenarzt 31: 145–149.

BAY E. (1964) *Principles of classification and their influence on our concepts of aphasia*. In DEREUCK A. V. S., O'CONNOR M. (eds.) *Disorders of language*. Boston, Little, Brown, and Company: 137–138.

BENSON D., WEIR W. (1972) *Acalculia: Acquired anarithmetia*. Cortex 8: 465–472.

BENSON F., GESCHWIND N. (1969) *The alexias*. In VINKEN P., BRUYN G. (eds.) *Handbook of clinical neurology 4*. Amsterdam, North Holland Publishing Company: 112–140.

BENTON A. (1967) *Constructional apraxia and the minor hemisphere*. Confinia Neurologica 29: 1–16.

BERGER H. (1911) *Über einen mit Schreibstörungen einhergehenden Krankheitsfall*. Monatszeitschrift für Psychiatrie und Neurologie 29: 357–366.

BERGER H. (1926) *Über Rechenstörungen bei Herderkrankungen des Grosshirns*. Archiv für Psychiatrie und Nervenkrankheiten 78: 238–263.

BERGES J. (1966) *Les dyspraxies chez l'enfant de 5 à 15 ans. Diagnostic. Conduite à tenir*. Revue de Neuropsychiatrie Infantile et d'Hygiène Mentale de l'Enfance 14: 267–276.

BERINGER K., STEIN J. (1930) *Analyse eines Falles von "reiner" Alexie*. Zeitschrift für Neurologie 123: 472–478.

176

BERTHA H. (1942–43) *Spiegelschrift der linken Hand.* Zeitschrift für die gesamte Neurologie und Psychiatrie 175: 68–96.

BEVER T., CHIARELLO R. (1974) *Cerebral dominance in musicians and nonmusicians.* Science 185: 537–539.

BIRCH H., LEE J. (1955) *Cortical inhibition in expressive aphasia.* Archives of Neurology and Psychiatry 74: 514–517.

BLACK J. (1951) *The effect of delayed sidetone upon vocal rate and intensity.* Journal of Speech and Hearing Disorders 16: 56–60.

BLUMSTEIN S., COOPER W. (1974) *Hemispheric processing of intonation contours.* Cortex 10: 146–158.

BLUMSTEIN S., GOODLASS H. (1972) *The perception of stress as a semantic cue in aphasia.* Journal of Speech and Hearing Research 15: 800–806.

BODAMER J. (1947) *Die Prosopagnosie.* Archiv für Psychiatrie und Nervenkrankheiten 179: 6–54.

BOETTIGER A. (1922) *Ein Fall von reiner motorischer Agraphie.* Archiv für Psychiatrie und Nervenkrankheiten 65: 87–103.

BOGEN J., GORDON H. (1971) *Musical tests for functional lateralization with intracarotid amobarbital.* Nature 230: 524–525.

BOLLER F., GREEN E. (1972) *Comprehension in severe aphasia.* Cortex 8: 382–394.

BOLLER F., MARCIE P. (1978) *Possible role of abnormal auditory feedback in conduction aphasia.* Neuropsychologia 16: 521–523.

BOLLER F., VRTUNSKI P., KIM Y., MACK J. (1978) *Delayed auditory feedback and aphasia.* Cortex 14: 212–226.

BOONE D. R. (1967) *A plan for rehabilitation of aphasic patients.* Archives of Physical Medicine and Rehabilitation 48: 410–414.

BOTEZ M., CALCAIANU G. (1961) *Etudes cliniques concernant les particularités de l'aphasie chez les gauchers.* Žurnal Nevropatologi i Psichiatril Imeni S.S. Korsakova 61: 820–828.

BOTEZ M., CRIGHEL E. (1971) *Partial disconnexion syndrome in an ambidextrous patient.* Brain 94: 487–494.

BOTEZ M., WERTHEIM N. (1959) *Expressive aphasia and amusia (following right frontal lesion in a right handed man).* Brain 82: 186–202.

BOUCHER M., MICHEL F., TOMMASI M., SCHOTT B. (1975) *Alexie sans agraphie.* In MICHEL F., SCHOTT B. *Les syndromes de disconnexion calleuse chez l'homme.* Lyon: 371–379.

BOUDOURESQUE J., PONCET M., SEBAHOUN M., ALICHERIF A. (1972) *Deux cas d'alexie sans agraphie avec troubles de la dénomination des couleurs et des images.* Oto-Neuro-Ophtalmologie 44: 297–304.

BRAIN R. (1961) *Speech disorders.* London, Butterworth.

BRAMWELL B. (1897) *Illustrative cases of aphasia.* Lancet 75 (March 27): 868–871.

BRESSON F., DE SCHONEN S., TZORTZIS E. (1972) *Etudes des perturbations dans les performances logico-arithmétiques chez des sujets atteints de diverses lésions cérébrales.* Langage 7: 108–122.

BRISSAUD E. (1894) *Sur l'aphasie d'articulation et l'aphasie d'intonation; à propos d'un cas d'aphasie motrice corticale sans agraphie.* Semaine Médicale 43: 341.

BRISSAUD E. (1901) *Aphasie d'articulation sans aphasie d'intonation.* Revue Neurologique: 666–669.

BRODAL A. (1973) *Self-observations and neuro-anatomical considerations after a stroke.* Brain 96: 675–694.

BURGER-PRINZ H. (1935) *Über eine Störung des Rechnens.* Der Nervenarzt 8: 586–589.

BYCHOWSKI Z. (1909) *Beiträge zur Nosographie der Apraxie.* Monatszeitschrift für Psychiatrie und Neurologie 26: Ergänzungsheft.

CAPLAN L., HEDLEY-WHYTE T. (1974) *Cuing and memory dysfunction in alexia without agraphia.* Brain 97: 251–262.

CARAMAZZA A., GORDON J., ZURIF E., DELUCA D. (1976) *Right-hemispheric damage and verbal problem solving behavior.* Brain and Language 3: 41–46.

CAREY S., DIAMOND R. (1977) *From piecemeal to configurational representation of faces,* Science 195: 312–314.

CARMON A., NACHSON I. (1973) *Ear asymmetry in perception of emotional non verbal stimuli.* Acta Psychologica 37: 351–357.

CHARBONNEAU G., RISSET J. (1975) *Différences entre oreille droite et oreille gauche pour la perception de la hauteur des sons.* Comptes rendus de l'Académie des Sciences, Paris, 281 (D): 163–167.

CHERRY E. (1953) *Some experiments on the recognition of speech with one and with two ears.* The Journal of the Acoustical Society of America, 25: 975–979.

COHEN D., SALANGA V., HULLY W., STEINBERG M., HARDY R. (1976) *Alexia without agraphia.* Neurology 26: 455–459.

COHN R. (1961) *Dyscalculia.* Archives of Neurology 4: 301–307.

COLLIGNON R., LECLERCQ C., MAHY J. (1977) *Etude de la sémiologie des troubles de calcul observés au cours des lésions corticales.* Acta Neurologica Belgica 77: 257–275.

CONRAD K. (1932–33) *Versuch einer psychologischen Analyse des Parietalsyndroms.* Monatsschrift für Psychiatrie und Neurologie 84: 28–97.

CONRAD K. (1948) *Strukturanalysen hirnpathologischer Fälle. Über den Gestaltwechsel der Sprachstörung bei einem Fall von corticaler motorischer Aphasie.* Archiv für Psychiatrie und Nervenkrankheiten, vereinigt mit Zeitschrift für die gesamte Neurologie und Psychiatrie 118/179: 502–567.

CONRAD K. (1948) *Strukturanalysen hirnpathologischer Fälle. Über die Broca'sche motorische Aphasie.* Deutsche Zeitschrift für Nervenheilkunde 159: 132–187.

CONRAD K. (1948) *Strukturanalysen hirnpathologischer Fälle. Zum Problem der Leitungsaphasie.* Deutsche Zeitschrift für Nervenheilkunde 159: 188–228.

CONRAD K. (1949) *Über aphasische Sprachstörungen bei hirnverletzten Linkshändern.* Der Nervenarzt 20: 148–154.

178

CONRAD K. (1953) *Hat der Begriff der "Leitungsstörung" in der Hirn-pathologie noch eine Berechtigung? Bemerkungen zu einer Arbeit von Leonhard.* Archiv für Psychiatrie und Nervenkrankheiten 190: 389–393.

CREMIEUX A., BOURDOURESQUES J., TAROSSIAN A., KAHLIF R., BILLE J. (1961) *Apraxie constructive. Troubles spatiaux gnostiques avec illusions microtéléopsiques. Infiltration glioblastique du carrefour pariéto-occipital droit, du splenium et du lobe occipital gauche.* Revue Neurologique 104: 66–75.

CRITCHLEY M. (1939) *The language of gesture.* New York, Haskell House Publishers.

CRITCHLEY M. (1953) *The parietal lobes.* London, Arnold.

CRITCHLEY M. (1964) *The problem of visual agnosia.* Journal of the Neurological Sciences 1: 274–290.

CRITCHLEY M. (1970) *Aphasiology.* Baltimore, Williams and Wilkins Company.

CROUZON, VALENCE (1923) *Un cas d'alexie pure.* Semaine des Hôpitaux de Paris 47: 1145–1149.

DAMASIO A., LIMA A., DAMASIO H. (1975) *Nervous function after right hemispherectomy.* Neurology 25: 89–93.

DARWIN C. (1975) *On the dynamic use of prosody in speech perception.* In COHEN A., NOOTEBOOM S. (eds.) *Structure and process in speech perception.* Heidelberg, Springer: 178–193.

DAVIS N., LEACH E. (1972) *Scaling aphasics' error responses.* Journal of Speech and Hearing Disorders 37: 305–313.

DAX M. (1865) *Lésions de la moitié gauche de l'encéphale coïncidant avec l'oubli des signes de la pensée.* Gazette Hebdomadaire de Médecine et de Chirurgie 33, 227: 260–262.

DEJERINE J. (1892) *Contribution à l'étude anatomopathologique et clinique des différentes variétés de cécité verbale.* Mémoires de la Société de Biologie 4: 61–90.

DEJERINE J. (1914) *Sémiologie des affections du système nerveux.* Paris, Masson.

DELATTRE P. (1966) *Des dix intonations de base du français.* The French Review, 40: 1–14.

DENNIS M., KOHN B. (1975) *Comprehension of syntax in infantile hemiplegics after cerebral hemidecortication: Left-hemisphere superiority.* Brain and Language 2: 472–482.

DENNIS M., WHITAKER H. (1976) *Language acquisition following hemidecortication. Linguistic superiority of the left over the right hemisphere.* Brain and Language 3: 404–433.

DENNIS M., WHITAKER H. (1977) *Hemispheric equipotentiality and language acquisition.* In SEGALOWITZ S., GRUBER F. (eds.) *Language development and neurological theory.* New York, Academic Press: 93–106.

DE RENZI E., PIECZURO A., VIGNOLO L. (1966) *Oral apraxia and aphasia.* Cortex 2: 50–73.

179

DE RENZI E., PIECZURO A., VIGNOLO L. (1968) *Ideational apraxia: A quantitative study.* Neuropsychologia 6: 41–52.

DIAMOND R., CAREY S. (1977) *Developmental changes in the representation of faces.* Journal of Experimental Child Psychology 23: 1–22.

DIDE M. (1938) *Les désorientations temporo-pariétales et la préponderance de l'hémisphère droit dans les agnoso-akinésies proprioceptives.* Encéphale 33: 276–295.

DOEHRING D., BARTHOLOMEUS B. (1971) *Laterality effects in voice recognition.* Neuropsychologia 9: 425–430.

DOEHRING D., ROSS R. (1972) *Voice recognition by matching to sample.* Journal of Psycholinguistic Research 1: 233–242.

DOMNICK O. (1943) *Gesichtsapraxie. Ein hirnpathologisches Syndrom, zugleich ein Beitrag zur Frage der rechtshirnigen Sprachstörung.* Deutsche Zeitschrift für Nervenheilkunde 155: 201–263.

DORDAIN E., DEGOS J., DORDAIN G. (1971) *Troubles de la voix dans les hémiplégies gauches.* Revue de Laryngologie 92: 178–188.

DUBOIS J., HECAEN H., MARCIE P. (1969) *L'agraphie "pure".* Neuropsychologica 7: 271–286.

DUBOIS-CHARLIER F. (1971) *Approche neurolinguistique du problème de l'alexie pure.* Journal de Psychologie Normale et Pathologique: 39–68.

DUENSING F. (1953) *Raumagnostische und ideatorisch-appraktische Störung des gestaltenden Handelns.* Deutsche Zeitschrift für Nervenheilkunde 170: 72–84.

DUFFY R., DUFFY J., PEARSON K. (1975) *Pantomime recognition in aphasics.* Journal of Speech and Hearing Research 18: 115–132.

DUVOIR J., BERTRAND I. (1935) *Hémiplégie gauche accompagnée, chez un droitier, de signes cliniques d'aphasie avec grosse prédominance d'agraphie. Ramollissement du corps calleux.* Bulletin de la société Médicale des Hôpitaux de Paris III, 51: 1071–1080.

EHRENWALD H. (1931) *Störung der Zeitauffassung, der räumlichen Orientierung, des Zeichnens und des Rechnens bei einem Hirnverletzten.* Zeitschrift für die gesamte Neurologie und Psychiatrie 132: 518–569.

EISENBURG A., SMITH R. (1971) *Nonverbal communication.* New York, Bobbs-Merrill.

EISENSON J. (1954) *Examining for aphasia.* New York, Psychological Corporation.

EISENSON J. (1962) *Language and intellectual modifications associated with right cerebral lesion.* Language and Speech 5: 49–53.

EISENSON J. (1973) *Adult aphasia: assessment and treatment.* New York, Appleton-Century-Crofts.

ERBSLOH J. (1903) *Über einen Fall von isolierter Agraphie und amnestischer Erinnerungsunfähigkeit.* Neurologisches Centralblatt 22: 1053–1060.

ETTLINGER E. (1965) *Functions of the corpus callosum.* London, Churchill.

180

FINCHAM R., NIBBELINK D., ASCHENBRENNER C. (1975) *Alexia with left homonymous hemianopia without agraphia.* Neurology 25: 1164–1168.

FONAGY I. (1976) *La vive voix: dynamique et changement.* Journal de Psychologie Normale et Pathologique 3–4: 275–304.

FORDYCE W., JONES R. H. (1966) *The efficacy of oral and pantomimed instruction for hemiplegic patients.* Archives of Physical Medicine and Rehabilitation 46: 676–680.

FRANCO L. (1977) personal communication.

FRANCO L., SPERRY R. (1977) *Hemisphere lateralization for cognitive processing of geometry.* Neuropsychologia 15: 107–113.

FREDERIKS J. (1963) *Constructional apraxia and cerebral dominance.* Psychiatria, Neurologia, Neurochirurgia 66: 522–530.

FRIEDLANDER B. (1968) *The effect of speaker identity, voice inflection, vocabulary and message redundancy on infants' selection of vocal reinforcement.* Journal of Experimental Child Psychology, 6: 443–459.

GALKOWSKI T. (1966) *Troubles de la parole de type aphasique chez les enfants (diagnostic et réhabilitation).* Acta Paedopsychiatrica 33: 245–251.

GARDNER H., LING P., FLAMM L., SILVERMAN J. (1975) *Comprehension and appreciation of humorous material following brain damage.* Brain 98: 399–412.

GAZZANIGA M., BOGEN J., SPERRY R. (1967) *Dyspraxia following division of the cerebral commissures.* Archives of Neurology 16: 606–612.

GAZZANIGA M., HILLYARD A. (1971) *Language and speech capacity of the right hemisphere.* Neuropsychologia 9: 273–280.

GAZZANIGA M. S., SPERRY R. W. (1967) *Language after section of the cerebral commissures.* Brain 90: 131–148.

GERSTMANN J. (1924) *Fingeragnosie: Eine umschriebene Störung der Orientierung am eigenen Körper.* Wiener klinische Wochenschrift 37: 1010–1012.

GERSTMANN J. (1927) *Fingeragnosie und isolierte Agraphie – ein neues Syndrom.* Zeitschrift für Psychiatrie 108: 152–177.

GERSTMANN J. (1957) *Some notes on the Gerstmann syndrome.* Neurology 7: 866–869.

GESCHWIND N. (1962) *The anatomy of acquired disorders of reading.* In MONEY J. *Reading disability.* Baltimore, Johns Hopkins University Press: 115–129.

GESCHWIND N. (1965) *Disconnexion syndromes in animals and man.* Brain 88: 237–294; 585–644.

GESCHWIND N. (1967) *Brain mechanisms suggested by studies of hemispheric connections.* In MILLIKAN C., DARLEY F. (eds.) *Brain mechanisms underlying speech and language.* New York, Grune & Stratton: 103–107.

GESCHWIND N., FUSILLO M. (1966) *Color-naming defects in association with alexia.* Archives of Neurology 15: 137–146.

GESCHWIND N., KAPLAN E. (1962) *A human cerebral deconnection syndrome.* Neurology 12: 675–685.

GIMENO A. (1969) *Apraxia ideomotriz.* Revista de Psiquiatria y Psicologia Médica de Europa y América Latinas 9: 221–243.

GLONING K. (1965) *Die cerebral bedingten Störungen des räumlichen Sehens und des Raumerlebens.* Wien, Maudrich.

GLONING I., GLONING K., SEITELBERGER F., TSCHABITSCHER H. (1955) *Ein Fall von reiner Wortblindheit mit Obduktionsbefund.* Wiener Zeitschrift für Nervenheilkunde 12: 194–215.

GOLDSTEIN K. (1910) *Über die amnestische Form der apraktischen Agraphie.* Neurologisches Centralblatt 29: 1252–1255.

GOLDSTEIN K. (1911) *Die amnestische und die zentrale Aphasie (Leitungsaphasie).* Archiv für Psychiatrie und Nervenkrankheiten 48: 314–343.

GOLDSTEIN K. (1914) *Ein Beitrag zur Lehre von der Bedeutung der Insel für die Sprache und der linken Hemisphäre für das linksseitige Tasten.* Archiv für Psychiatrie und Nervenkrankheiten 55: 158–173.

GOLDSTEIN K. (1948) *Language and language disturbances.* New York, Grune and Stratton.

GOLLNITZ G. (1958) *Beitrag zum Problem der motorischen Hörstummheit.* Archiv für Psychiatrie und Nervenkrankheiten 197: 77–82.

GOODGLASS H., FODOR I., SCHULHOFF C. (1967) *Prosodic factors in grammar – Evidence from aphasia.* Journal of Speech and Hearing Research 10: 5–20.

GOODGLASS H., KAPLAN E. (1963) *Disturbance of gesture and pantomime in aphasia.* Brain 86: 703–720.

GOODGLASS H., KAPLAN E. (1972) *The assessment of aphasia and related disorders.* Philadelphia, Lea and Febiger.

GOODGLASS H., QUADFASEL F. (1954) *Language laterality in left handed aphasics.* Brain 77: 521–548.

GORDON H., BOGEN J. (1974) *Hemispheric lateralization of singing after intracarotid sodium amylobarbitone.* Journal of Neurology, Neurosurgery and Psychiatry 37: 727–738.

GOTT P. (1973) *Cognitive abilities following right and left hemispherectomy.* Cortex 9: 266–274.

GREEN G., BOLLER F. (1974) *Features of auditory comprehension in severely impaired aphasics.* Cortex 10: 133–145.

GREENBLATT S. (1973) *Alexia without agraphia or hemianopia: Anatomical analysis of an autopsied case.* Brain 96: 307–316.

GRENIER D. (1969) *La prosopagnosie et l'agnosie de la voix.* Montreal, unpublished thesis.

GREWEL F. (1969) *The acalculias.* In VINKEN P., BRUYN G. (eds.) *Handbook of clinical neurology* 4, Amsterdam, North-Holland Publishing Company: 181–194.

GRIFFITH H., DAVIDSON M. (1966) *Long-term changes in intellect and behaviour after hemispherectomy.* Journal of Neurology, Neurosurgery and Psychiatry 29: 571–576.

GRÜNBAUM A. (1930) *Über Apraxie.* Zentralblatt für die gesamte Neurologie und Psychiatrie 55: 788–792.

182

HAGGARD M., PARKINSON A. (1971) *Stimulus and task factors as determinants of ear advantages.* Quarterly Journal of Experimental Psychology, 23: 168–177.

HARTL J. (1964) *Motorische Aphasie und Apraxie.* Acta Universitatis Palackianae Olomucensis 34: 217–221.

HASAERTS-VAN GEERTRUYDEN E. (1966) *Contribution à l'étude de la dyspraxie faciale.* Revue de Neuropsychiatrie Infantile et d'Hygiène Mentale de l'Enfance 14: 731–741.

HEAD H. (1926) *Aphasia and kindred disorders of speech.* Cambridge, University Press.

HECAEN H. (1962) *Clinical symptomatology in right and left hemispheric lesions.* In MOUNTCASTLE V. (ed.) *Interhemispheric relations and cerebral dominance.* Baltimore, Johns Hopkins: 215–243.

HECAEN H. (1967) *Brain mechanisms suggested by studies of parietal lobe.* In MILLIKAN C., DARLEY F. (eds.) *Brain mechanisms underlying speech and language.* New York, Grune and Stratton: 146–166.

HECAEN H. (1969) *Aphasic, apraxic and agnostic syndromes in right and left hemisphere lesions.* In VINKEN P., BRUYN G. (eds.) *Handbook of clinical neurology* 4, Amsterdam, North-Holland Publishing Company: 291–311.

HECAEN H., AJURIAGUERRA J. (1963) *Les gauchers.* Paris, Presses Universitaires de France.

HECAEN H., AJURIAGUERRA J. (1964) *Le cortex cérébral. Etude neuropsycho-pathologique.* Paris, Masson.

HECAEN H., AJURIAGUERRA J., MASSONNET J. (1951) *Les troubles visuo-constructifs par lésion pariéto-occipitale droite. Rôle des perturbations vestibulaires.* Encéphale 40: 122–179.

HECAEN H., ANGELERGUES R. (1962) *L'aphasie, l'apraxie, l'agnosie chez les gauchers: Modalité et fréquence des troubles selon l'hémisphère atteint.* Revue Neurologique 106: 510–515.

HECAEN H., ANGELERGUES R. (1963) *La cécité psychique. Etude critique de la notion d'agnosie. A propos de 415 cas de lésions cérébrales hémisphériques postérieures, dont 102 avec agnosie optique.* Paris, Masson.

HECAEN H., ANGELERGUES R., HOULLIER S. (1961) *Les variétés cliniques des acalculies au cours des lésions rétrorolandiques: approche statistique du problème.* Revue Neurologique 105: 85–103.

HECAEN H., MARCIE P. (1967) *L'agraphie au cours de l'aphasie de conduction.* Wiener Zeitschrift für Nervenheilkunde und deren Grenzgebiete 25: 193–203.

HECAEN H., PENFIELD W., BERTRAND C., MALMO R. (1956) *The syndrome of apractognosia due to lesions of the minor cerebral hemisphere.* Archives of Neurology and Psychiatry 75: 400–434.

HEILMAN K. (1973) *A tapping test in apraxia.* Neurology 23: 400–405.

HEILMAN K. (1973) *Ideational apraxia – A re-definition.* Brain 96: 861–864.

183

HEILMAN K. (1974) Untitled paper presented at the symposium "Experimental approaches to Aphasia". Annual meeting of the International Neuropsychological Society, Boston, Ma, February 7, 1974.

HEILMAN K., COYLE J., GONYEA E., GESCHWIND N. (1973) *Apraxia and agraphia in a left-hander.* Brain 96: 21–28.

HEILMAN K., SCHOLES R., WATSON R. (1975) *Auditory affective agnosia.* Journal of Neurology, Neurosurgery, and Psychiatry 38: 69–72.

HENSCHEN S. (1920) *Klinische und anatomische Beiträge zur Pathologie des Gehirns.* 5. Teil: *Über Aphasie, Amusie, Akalkulie.* (1920) 6. Teil: *Über die sensorische Aphasie.* (1922) 7. Teil: *Über motorische Aphasie und Agraphie.* Stockholm, Nordiska.

HENSCHEN S. (1926) *On the function of the right hemisphere of the brain in relation to the left hemisphere in speech, music and calculation.* Brain 49: 110–123.

HENSCHEN S. (1927) *Zur Lokalisierung der Rechenfunktion.* Archiv für Psychiatrie und Nervenkrankheiten 79: 375–382.

HERRMANN G. (1928) *Beiträge zur Lehre von den Störungen des Rechnens bei Herderkrankungen des Occipitallappens (Alkalkulie Henschens).* Monatsschrift für Psychiatrie und Neurologie 70: 193–278.

HERRMANN G., PÖTZL O. (1926) *Über die Agraphie und ihre lokaldiagnostischen Beziehungen.* Beihefte Monatsschrift für Psychiatrie und Neurologie 35.

HEUYER G., FELD M. (1954) *Hémispherectomie gauche pour atrophie cicatricielle chez un enfant droitier. Discussion de l' acquisition postopératoire du langage.* Revue Neurologique 90: 52–58.

HINSHELWOOD J. (1902) *Four cases of word-blindness.* Lancet: 358–363.

HOEFT J. (1957) *Klinisch-anatomischer Beitrag zur Kenntnis der Nachsprechaphasie (Leitungsaphasie).* Deutsche Zeitschrift für Nervenheilkunde 175: 560–594.

HOFF H. (1954) *Die Rückbildung der Aphasie.* Münchner medizinische Wochenschrift 104: 92–113.

HOLMES G. (1950) *Pure word blindness.* Folia Psychiatrica, Neurologica et Neurochirurgia Neerlandica 53: 279–288.

JACKSON J. (1932) *Selected writings*, edited by J. TAYLOR. London, Hodder and Stoughton.

KERN A. (1932) *Der Einfluss des Hörens auf des Stottern.* Archiv für Psychiatrie und Nervenkrankheiten 97: 429–449.

KIM Y., BONSTELLE C., ROYER F., BOLLER F. (1979) *The efficacy of neuropsychological evaluation.* Paper read at the annual meeting of the International Neuropsychological Society, New York, NY, February 2, 1979.

KING F., KIMURA D. (1972) *Left ear superiority in dichotic perception of vocal nonverbal sounds.* Canadian Journal of Psychology 26: 111–115.

KINSBOURNE M., WARRINGTON E. (1962) *A study of finger agnosia.* Brain 85: 47–66.

KLEIST K. (1916) *Über Leitungsaphasie und grammatische Störungen.* Monatsschrift für Psychiatrie und Neurologie 40: 118–199.

KLEIST K. (1934) *Gehirnpathologie.* Leipzig, Barth.

KLING A. (1972) *Effects of amygdalectomy on social-affective behavior in nonhuman primates.* In ELEFTHERIO B. (ed.), *The neurology of the amygdala.* New York, Plenum Press: 511–536.

KOHLMEYER K. (1970) *Aphasie-Syndrome und hirnlokale Zirkulationsstörungen der dominanten Hemisphäre im Karotisangiogramm.* In LEISCHNER A. (ed.) *Die Rehabilitation der Aphasie in den romanischen Ländern nebst Beiträgen zur Aphasieforschung.* Stuttgart, Thieme: 59–70.

KONORSKI J. (1970) *Pathophysiological mechanisms of speech on the basis of studies on aphasia.* Acta Neurobiologiae Experimentalis 30: 189–210.

KRAMER F. (1917) *Reine Agraphie.* Neurologisches Centralblatt 36: 570–572.

KREINDLER A., IONASESCU V. (1961) *A case of pure word blindness.* Journal of Neurology, Neurosurgery and Psychiatry 24: 275–280.

KROLL M., STOLBUN D. (1933) *Was ist konstruktive Apraxie?* Zeitschrift für die gesamte Neurologie und Psychiatrie 148: 142–158.

LANGE J. (1930) *Fingeragnosie und Agraphie. (Eine psychopathologische Studie).* Monatsschrift für Psychiatrie und Neurologie 76: 129–188.

LANGE J. (1936) *Agnosien und Apraxien.* In BUMKE O., FÖRSTER O. (eds.) *Handbuch der Neurologie VI.* Berlin, Springer.

LANGE J., WAGNER W. (1938) *Kompensationsschritte bei Zerstörung des linken Occipitallapens durch einen Tumor.* Zeitschrift für die gesamte Neurologie und Psychiatrie 161: 199–204.

LARSEN B., SKINHOY E., LASSEN N. (1978) *Variations in regional cortical blood flow in the right and left hemispheres during automatic speech.* Brain 101: 193–209.

LASSEN N., INGVAR D., SKINHOY E. (1978) *Brain function and blood flow.* Scientific American 239, 4: 50–59.

LEATHERS D. (1976) *Nonverbal communication systems.* Boston, Allyn and Bacon, Inc.

LEBRUN Y. (1967) *Le phonème, unité d'emploi ou unité de description?* Revue Belge de Philologie et d'Histoire 45: 761–776.

LEBRUN Y. (1967) *Linguistic analysis of two cases of emissive aphasia.* Journal of the Neurological Sciences 4: 271–277.

LEBRUN Y. (1974) *Die unterwertige Hirnhälfte und die Sprache.* Der Nervenarzt 45: 510–513.

LEBRUN Y. (1976) *Neurolinguistic models of language and speech.* In WHITAKER H. (ed.) *Studies in neurolinguistics 1.* New York, Academic Press: 1–30.

LEBRUN Y., HOOPS R. (1974) *Intelligence and aphasia.* Amsterdam, Swets & Zeitlinger.

LEBRUN Y., LEBRUN N. (1971) *On the role of visual feedback in writing.* ITL 13: 59–62.

185

LEE B. (1950) *Effects of delayed speech feedback.* Journal of the Acoustic Society of America 22: 824–826.

LEHMANN-FACIUS H. (1951) *Differentialdiagnose konstruktiv-agraphischer und apraktischer Syndrome bei Tumoren des hinteren Scheitellappens.* Deutsche Zeitschrift für Nervenheilkunde 165: 142–164.

LEISCHNER A. (1969) *The agraphias.* In VINKEN P., BRUYN G. (eds.) *Handbook of clinical neurology* IV. Amsterdam, North-Holland Publishing Company: 141–180.

LEISCHNER A. (1970) *Die Rehabilitation der Aphasie in den romanischen Ländern nebst Beiträgen zur Aphasieforschung.* Stuttgart, Thieme.

LEONHARD K. (1939) *Die Bedeutung optisch-räumlicher Vorstellungen für das elementaire Rechnen.* Zeitschrift für die gesamte Neurologie und Psychiatrie 164: 321–351.

LEONHARD K. (1940) *Vorstellungstypen des elementaren Rechnens.* Zeitschrift für angewandte Psychologie 58: 193–212.

LEONHARD K. (1952a) *Reine Agraphie und konstruktive Apraxie als Ausdruck einer Leitungsstörung.* Archiv für Psychiatrie und Nervenkrankheiten 188: 471–503.

LEONHARD K. (1952b) *Entstehung reiner Agraphien durch rechtsseitige Hirnherde.* Deutsche Zeitschrift für Nervenheilkunde 169: 111–122.

LEONHARD K. (1952c) *Rechen- und zeitliche Orientierungsstörung bei Agraphie und konstruktiver Apraxie.* Archiv für Psychiatrie und Nervenkrankheiten 188: 504–510.

LEONHARD K. (1953) *Zur Frage der Leitungsstörung in der Gehirnpathologie.* Archiv für Psychiatrie und Nervenkrankheiten 190: 466–468.

LEONHARD K. (1954) *Innervatorische und ideokinetische Form motorischer Aphasie.* Der Nervenarzt 25: 177–186.

LEONHARD K. (1956) *Apraxie der Blickbewegungen mit konstruktiver Apraxie und reiner Agraphie.* Archiv für Psychiatrie und Nervenkrankheiten 195: 117–131.

LEONHARD K. (1962) *Das Bild der ideokinetischen Agraphie.* Deutsche Zeitschrift für Nervenheilkunde 183: 502–516.

LEONHARD K. (1965) *Über parietale Aphasie.* Psychiatrie, Neurologie und medizinische Psychologie 17: 162–165.

LEONHARD K., NEUMANN H. (1957) *Verlust der Rechenkurve bei einem darstellenden Rechentypus.* Der Nervenarzt: 123–125.

LEONHARD K., SCHOTT G. (1960) *Über die Entstehung der Spiegelschrift der linken Hand.* Wiener Zeitschrift für Nervenheilkunde und deren Grenzgebiete 18: 246–252.

LEONHARD K., BERENDT H., LINDNER A. (1968) *Motorische Hörstummheit und parietale Aphasie. Zugleich eine Frage nach der Plastizität des Gehirns.* Journal of the Neurological Sciences 5: 511–517.

LEVINE D., CALVANIO R. (1978) *A study of the visual defect in alexia – simultanagnosia.* Brain 101: 65–82.

LEWANDOWSKY M. (1911) *Rechtshirnigkeit bei einem Rechtshänder.* Zeitschrift für die gesamte Neurologie und Psychiatrie 4: 211–216.

LEWANDOWSKY M., STADELMANN E. (1908) *Uber einen bemerkenswerten Fall von Hirnblutung und über Rechenstörungen bei Herderkrankung des Gehirns.* Journal für Psychologie und Neurologie (Leipzig) 11: 249–265.

LHERMITTE J. (1968) *Les fondements anatomiques de la latéralité.* In KOURILSKY R., GRAPIN P. (eds.) *Main droite et main gauche.* Paris, Presses Universitaires de France: 5–24.

LHERMITTE F., BEAUVOIS M. (1973) *A visual-speech disconnexion syndrome – Report of a case with optic aphasia, agnosic alexia and colour agnosia.* Brain 96: 695–714.

LHERMITTE F., GAUTIER I. (1969) *Aphasias.* In VINKEN P., BRUYN W. (eds.) *Handbook of clinical neurology* IV. Amsterdam, North-Holland Publishing Company: 84–104.

LHERMITTE J., MOUZON J. (1941) *Sur l'apractognosie géométrique et l'apraxie constructive consécutives aux lésions du lobe occipital.* Revue Neurologique 73: 415–431.

LHERMITTE J., TRELLES J. (1933) *Sur l'apraxie pure constructive. Les troubles de la pensée spatiale et de la somatognosie dans l'apraxie.* Encéphale 28: 413–444.

LIEPMANN H. (1900) *Das Krankheitsbild der Apraxie (motorische Asymbolie).* Monatsschrift für Psychiatrie und Neurologie 8: 15–44, 102–132, 182–197.

LIEPMANN H. (1905) *Über Störungen des Handelns bei Gehirnkranken.* Berlin, Karger.

LIEPMANN H. (1905) *Der weitere Krankheitsverlauf bei dem einseitig Apraktischen und der Gehirnbefund auf Grund von Serienschnitten.* Monatsschrift für Psychiatrie und Neurologie 17: 289–311.

LIEPMANN H. (1908) *Drei Aufsätze aus dem Apraxiegebiet.* Berlin, Karger.

LIEPMANN H. (1913) *Motorische Aphasie und Apraxie.* Monatsschrift für Psychiatrie und Neurologie 34: 485–495.

LIEPMANN H. (1929) *Klinische und psychologische Untersuchung und anatomischer Befund bei einem Fall von Dyspraxie und Agraphie.* Monatsschrift für Psychiatrie und Neurologie 71: 169–214.

LIEPMANN H., MAAS O. (1907) *Fall von linksseitiger Agraphie und Apraxie bei rechtsseitiger Lähmung.* Journal für Psychologie und Neurologie 10: 214–227.

LIEPMANN H., PAPPENHEIM M. (1914) *Über einen Fall von sogenannter Leitungsaphasie mit anatomischem Befund.* Zeitschrift für die gesamte Neurologie und Psychiatrie 27: 1–41.

LINDQVIST T. (1935) *De l'acalculie.* Acta Medica Scandinavica 37: 225–271.

LINDQVIST T. (1936) *Nouvelles études sur le problème de l'acalculie.* Acta Medica Scandinavica 38: 217–277.

LURIA A. (1964) *Factors and forms of aphasia.* In DE REUCK A., O'CONNOR M. (eds.) *Disorders of language.* London, Churchill: 143–161.

LURIA A. (1965) *Aspects of aphasia.* Journal of the Neurological Sciences 2: 278–287.

187

LURIA A. (1966) *Higher cortical functions in man.* London, Tavistock Publications.

LURIA A., TSVETKOVA L. (1967) *Les troubles de la résolution des problèmes.* Paris, Gauthier-Villars.

MANN V., DIAMOND R., CAREY S. (1977) *Voice discrimination in children aged six to ten.* Cambridge, M.I.T. Psychology Department.

MARCIE P., HECAEN H., DUBOIS J., ANGELERGUES R. (1965) *Les réalisations du langage chez les malades atteints de lésions de l'hémisphère droit.* Neuropsychologia 3: 217–245.

MARIE P. (1906) *Que faut-il penser des aphasies sous corticales?* La Semaine Médicale 26: 493–500.

MARINESCO G., GRIGORESCO D., AXENTE S. (1938) *Considérations sur l'aphasie croisée.* Encéphale 33: 27–46.

MARTIN B. (1962) *Communicative aids for the adult aphasic.* Springfield, Ill., Charles C. Thomas.

MARTIN P. (1954) *Pure world blindness as a disturbance of visual space perception.* Proceedings of the Royal Society of Medicine 47: 293–295.

MAYER-GROSS W. (1935) *Some observations of apraxia.* Proceedings of the Royal Society of Medicine 28: 1203–1212.

MAYER-GROSS W. (1936) *The question of visual impairment in constructional apraxia.* Proceedings of the Royal Society of Medicine 29: 1396–1400.

MAYER-GROSS W. (1936) *Further observations on apraxia.* The Journal of Mental Sciences 82: 744–762.

McFIE J. (1961) *The effect of hemispherectomy on intellectual functioning in cases of infantile hemiplegia.* Journal of Neurology, Neurosurgery and Psychiatry 24: 240–249.

McFIE J., ZANGWILL O. (1960) *Visual constructive disabilities associated with lesions of the left cerebral hemisphere.* Brain 83: 243–260.

MECHROTA A., ANKLESARIA J., KHOSLA S. (1964) *Congenital ocular motor apraxia.* Neurology India 12: 144–148.

MEHLER J., BARRIERE M., JASSIK-GERSCHFELD D. (1976) *La reconnaissance de la voix maternelle par le nourrisson.* La Recherche 70: 786–788.

MEYER S. (1908) *Apraktische Agraphie bei einem Rechtshirner.* Zentralblatt für Nervenheilkunde und Psychiatrie 31: 673–678.

MEYER S. (1908) *Relative Eupraxie bei Rechtsgelähmten.* Deutsche medizinische Wochenschrift 34: 1143–1145.

MICHAUX J., LAMACHE, PICARD (1924) *Alexie pure à début brusque suivie d'ictus passager avec hémorragie méningée.* Semaine des Hôpitaux de Paris 48: 1703–1706.

MILLIKAN C., DARLEY F. (1967) *Brain mechanisms underlying speech and language.* New York, Grune and Stratton.

MILNER B. (1962) *Laterality effects in audition.* In MOUNTCASTLE V. (ed.) *Interhemispheric relations and cerebral dominance.* Baltimore, Johns Hopkins Press: 177–195.

MILNER B. (1974) *Hemispheric specialization: Scope and limits*. In SCHMITT F., WORDEN F. (eds.), *The Neurosciences. Third study program*. Cambridge, M.I.T. Press: 75–89.

MONRAD-KROHN H. H. (1947) *Dysprosody or altered "melody of language"*. Brain, 70: 405–415.

MULLER D. (1968) *Neurologische Untersuchung und Diagnostik im Kindesalter*. Wien, Springer.

NAESER M., HAYWARD R., ZATZ L. (1976) *Correlation between CT scan findings and Boston Diagnostic Aphasia Examination*. Paper read, at the Academy of Aphasia, 14th Annual Meeting, Miami, Fl, October 12, 1976.

NIELSEN J. (1946) *Agnosia, apraxia, aphasia*. New York, Hoeber.

NIESSL VON, MAYENDORF E. (1930) *Vom Lokalisationsproblem der artikulierten Sprache*. Leipzig, Barth.

NIESSL VON, MAYENDORF E. (1933) *Beiträge zur Aphasielehre*. Zentralblatt für die gesamte Neurologie und Psychiatrie 65: 184–185.

NIESSL VON, MAYENDORF E. (1933) *Zur Frage der sogenannten parietalen Aphasie*. Zeitschrift für die gesamte Neurologie und Psychiatrie 147: 1–49.

OMBREDANE A. (1944) *Etude de psychologie médicale*. Rio de Janeiro, Atlantica Editora.

OPPENHEIM H. (1908) *Lehrbuch der Nervenkrankheiten*. Berlin, Karger (5th edition).

OSGOOD C., MIRON M. (1963) *Approaches to the study of aphasia*. Urbana, University of Illinois Press.

PATERSON A., ZANGWILL O. (1944) *Disorders of visual space perception associated with lesions of the right cerebral hemisphere*. Brain 67: 331–358.

PELZ A. (1912) *Zur Lehre von den transcorticalen Aphasien*. Zeitschrift für die gesamte Neurologie und Psychiatrie 11: 110–152.

PELZ A. (1913) *Zwei Fälle von apraktischer Agraphie*. Zeitschrift für die gesamte Neurologie und Psychiatrie 19: 540–576.

PENFIELD W., ROBERTS L. (1959) *Speech and brain mechanisms*. Princeton, University Press.

PERITZ G. (1918) *Zur Pathopsychologie des Rechnens*. Deutsche Zeitschrift für Nervenheilkunde 61: 234–240.

PERON N., GOUTNER V. (1944) *Alexie pure sans hémianopsie*. Revue Neurologique 76: 81–82.

PFEIFER R. (1922) *Die rechte Hemisphäre und das Handeln*. Zeitschrift für die gesamte Neurologie und Psychiatrie 77: 471–508.

PICK A. (1898) *Beiträge zur Pathologie und pathologischen Anatomie des Zentralnervensystems*. Berlin, Karger.

PICK A. (1913) *Die agrammatischen Sprachstörungen*. Berlin, Springer.

PICK A. (1973) *Aphasia*. Springfield, Ill., Charles C. Thomas.

PICKETT L. (1972) *An assessment of gestural and pantomimic deficit in*

189

aphasic patients. Unpublished master's thesis, University of New Mexico.

PIERCY M., HECAEN H., AJURIAGUERRA J. (1960) *Constructional apraxia associated with unilateral cerebral lesions, left and right sided cases compared*. Brain 83: 225–242.

PIERCY M., SMYTH V. (1962) *Right hemisphere dominance for certain nonverbal intellectual skills*. Brain 85: 775–790.

POECK K., KERSCHENSTEINER M. (1971) *Ideomotor apraxia following right-sided cerebral lesion in a left-handed subject*. Neuropsychologia 9: 359–361.

POGGI, G. (1968) *Considerazioni sintetice sulle aprassie motoric facio-bucco-linguali.* Folia Neuropsychiatrica 11: 83–102.

POLLACK I., PICKETT J., SUMBY W. (1954) *On the identification of speakers by voice*. The Journal of the Acoustical Society of America 26: 403–406.

POPPELREUTER W. (1917 and 1918) *Die psychischen Schädigungen durch Kopfschuss im Kriege 1914/17*. Vol. 1 and 2. Leipzig, Voss.

PORCH B. (1967) *Porch Index of Communicative Ability*. Palo Alto, Calif., Consulting Psychologists Press (Volumes I and II).

PORCH B. (1971) *Multidimensional scoring in aphasia testing*. Journal of Speech and Hearing Research 14: 776–792.

POTTS C. (1901) *Ein Fall von vorübergehender motorischer Aphasie mit kompletter Anomie, fast kompletter Agraphie und Vollblindheit*. American Medical Association 18: 1239–1241.

PÖTZL O. (1925) *Über die parietal bedingte Aphasie und ihren Einfluss auf das Sprechen mehrerer Sprachen*. Zeitschrift für die gesamte Neurologie und Psychiatrie 96: 100–124.

REICHARDT M. (1918) *Allgemeine und spezielle Psychiatrie*. (2nd edition) Jena, Fischer.

RICHTER H. (1962) *Zur Frage der ideokinetischen Form der motorischen Aphasie*. Deutsche Zeitschrift für Nervenheilkunde 183: 484–501.

RICHTER H. (1965) *Verlaufsbeobachtungen über längere Zeit bei ideokinetischer motorischer Aphasie*. Deutsche Zeitschrift für Nervenheilkunde 187: 58–62.

RIEGER C. (1909) *Über Apraxie in dem Hirn*. Jena, Fischer.

RIESE W. (1949) *Aphasia in brain tumors*. Confinia Neurologica 9: 64–79.

ROBERTS H. (1958) *Functional plasticity in cortical speech areas and integration of speech*. Archives of Neurology and Psychiatry 79: 275–283.

RUBENS A., BENSON F. (1971) *Associative visual agnosia*. Archives of Neurology 24: 305–316.

RUSSELL W., ESPIR M. (1961) *Traumatic aphasia*. Oxford, University Press.

SARKISSOW S. (1967) *Grundriss der Struktur und Funktion des Gehirns*. Berlin, Volk und Gesundheit.

190

SASANUMA S. (1974) *Kanji versus kana processing in alexia with transient agraphia: A case report.* Cortex 10: 89–97.

SARNO J., SWISHER C., SARNO M. (1969) *Aphasia in a congenitally deaf man.* Cortex 5: 398–414.

SCHAECHTER M. (1935) *A propos d'un cas d'aphasie croisée. Etude clinique.* Revue Médicale de la Suisse Romande 55: 947–950.

SCHELLER H. (1938) *Amnetische Aphasie, Wortblindheit und Störung des optischen Vorstellens.* Monatsschrift für Psychiatrie und Neurologie 100: 33–91.

SCHLANGER B., SCHLANGER P., GERSTMAN L. (1976) *The perception of emotionally toned sentences by right hemisphere damaged and aphasic subjects.* Brain and Language 3: 396–403.

SCHLANGER P. (1976) *Training the adult aphasic to pantomime.* Presentation at the American Speech and Hearing Convention, Houston, Texas.

SCHLANGER P., GEFFNER D., DiCARRADO C. (1974) *A comparison of gestural communication with aphasics: pre- and post-therapy.* Presentation at American Speech and Hearing Convention, Las Vegas, Nevada.

SCHLESINGER B. (1928) *Zur Auffassung der optischen und konstruktiven Apraxie.* Zeitschrift für die gesamte Neurologie und Psychiatrie 117: 649–697.

SCHÖNFELDER T. (1967) *Katamnestische Erhebungen bei hörstummen Kindern.* Jahrbuch für Jugendpsychiatrie und ihre Grenzgebiete 5: 92–97.

SCHUELL H., JENKINS J., JIMENEZ-PABON J. (1964) *Aphasia in adults.* New York, Harper and Row.

SCHULZE H. (1959) *Die Notwendigkeit einer topistischen Aphasie-forschung und die Abhängigkeit der Rechenstörungen vom prämorbiden Rechentyp.* Psychiatrie, Neurologie und medizinische Psychologie 11: 50–57.

SCHULZE H. (1965) *Die klinische Analyse kombinierter hirnpathologischer Störungen (Aphasie, Apraxie, Agnosie).* Beiträge zur Neurochirurgie, Heft 9. Leipzig, Barth.

SCHULZE H. (1965) *Tumoren des Parietallappens.* In LEONHARD K. (ed.) *Die klinische Lokalisation der Hirntumoren in der Kritik der technischen, bioptischen und autoptischen Nachprüfung.*

SCHULZE H. (1966) *Architektonische Untersuchungen zur Frage der ideokinetischen motorischen Aphasie.* Journal für Hirnforschung 8: 111–127.

SEELERT H. (1920) *Beitrag zur Kenntnis der Rückbildung von Apraxie.* Monatsschrift für Psychiatrie und Neurologie 48: 125–149.

SEILER F. (1914) *Über einen Fall von reiner Agraphie bei einem an linksseitiger Hemiparese leidenden Linkshänder, bedingt durch einen Erweichungsherd im Gyrus supramarginalis dexter.* Neurologisches Zentralblatt 33: 311–312.

SINGER H., LOW A. (1933) *Acalculia.* Archives of Neurology and Psychiatry (Chicago) 29: 467–498.

SINGH S., SCHLANGER B. (1969) *Effects of delayed sidetone on the speech of aphasic, dysarthric and mentally retarded subjects*. Language and Speech 12: 167–174.

SITTIG O. (1921) *Störung des Ziffernschreibens und Rechnens bei einem Hirnverletzten*. Monatsschrift für Psychiatrie und Neurologie 49: 299–305.

SMITH A. (1966) *Speech and other functions after left (dominant) hemispherectomy*. Journal of Neurology, Neurosurgery and Psychiatry 29: 467–471.

SMITH A. (1972) *Dominant and nondominant hemispherectomy*. In SMITH W. (ed.) *Drugs, development and cerebral function*. Springfield, Thomas: 37–68.

SMITH A., BURKLUND C. (1966) *Dominant hemispherectomy*. Science 153: 1280–1282.

SMITH A., SUGAR O. (1975) *Development of above normal language and intelligence 21 years after left hemispherectomy*. Neurology 25: 813–818.

SMITH G. (1970) *A simplified guide to statistics*. New York, Holt, Rinehart, and Winston.

SPALDING J., ZANGWILL O. (1950) *Disturbance of number-form in a case of brain injury*. Journal of Neurology, Neurosurgery and Psychiatry 13: 24–29.

SPERRY R., GAZZANIGA M. (1967) *Language following surgical disconnection of the hemispheres*. In MILLIKAN C., DARLEY F. *Brain mechanisms underlying speech and language*. New York, Grune & Stratton: 108–121.

SPERRY R., GAZZANIGA M., BOGEN J. (1969) *Interhemispheric relationships. The neocortical commissures; syndromes of hemisphere disconnection*. In VINKEN P., BRUYN G. (eds.) *Handbook of clinical neurology 4*. Amsterdam, North-Holland Publishing Company: 273–290.

STANTON J. (1958) *The effects of DAF on the speech of aphasic patients*. Scottish Medical Journal 3: 378–384.

STACHOWIAK F., POECK K. (1976) *Functional disconnection in pure alexia and color naming deficit demonstrated by facilitating methods*. Brain and Language 3: 135–143.

STENGEL E., LODGE PATCH I. (1955) *"Central" aphasia associated with parietal symptoms*. Brain 78: 401–416.

STIER E. (1917) *Isolierte Agraphie und Alexie bei einem linksseitig gelähmten Linkshänder*. Neurologisches Zentralblatt 36: 92–93.

STOCKERT F. (1934) *Lokalisation und klinische Differenzierung des Symptoms der Nichtwahrnehmung einer Körperhälfte*. Deutsche Zeitschrift für Nervenheilkunde 134: 1–13.

STOCKERT F. (1934) *Das Gerstmannsche Syndrom der Fingeragnosie mit besonderer Berücksichtigung der Sprach- und Schreibstörung*. Monatsschrift für Psychiatrie und Neurologie 88: 121–151.

STOCKERT F. (1942) *Probleme der Hirnlokalisation mit besonderer Berück-*

sichtigung des Scheitelhirns. Fortschritte der Neurologie, Psychiatrie und ihrer Grenzgebiete 14: 46–68.

STOCKERT F. (1949) *Patho-physiologische Gesichtspunkte zur Hirnlokalisation.* Psychiatrie, Neurologie und medizinische Psychologie 1: 19–25.

STRAUSS H. (1924) *Über konstruktive Apraxie.* Monatsschrift für Psychiatrie und Neurologie 56: 65–124.

SUBIRANA A. (1958) *The prognosis in aphasia in relation to cerebral dominance and handedness.* Brain 81: 415–425.

TAUB J., TANGUAY P., DOUBLEDAY C., CLARKSON D., REMINGTON R. (1976) *Hemisphere and ear asymmetry in the auditory evoked response to musical chord stimuli.* Physiological Psychology, 4: 11–17.

THIELE R. (1928) *Aphasie, Apraxie, Agnosie.* In BUMKE O. (ed.) *Handbuch der Geisteskrankheiten.* Vol. 2, II. Berlin, Springer.

TISSOT R., LHERMITTE F., DUCARNE B. (1963) *Etat intellectuel des aphasiques. Essai d'une nouvelle approche à travers des épreuves perceptives et opératoires.* Encéphale 52: 285–320.

TOMKIEWICZ S. (1963) *L'aphasie chez l'enfant.* La Médecine Infantile 70: 509–516

TOMKIEWICZ S. (1964) *Aphasie chez l'enfant.* Revue de Neuropsychiatrie Infantile et d'Hygiène Mentale de l'Enfance 12: 109–122.

TZAVARAS A. (1967) *Contribution à l'étude de l'agnosie des physionomies.* Faculté de Médecine de Paris, thesis.

ULLMANN J. (1974) *Psychologie der Lateralität.* Bern, Huber.

VAN LANCKER D., FROMKIN V. (1973) *Hemispheric specialization for pitch and tone: Evidence from Thai.* Journal of Phonetics I: 101–109.

VINCENT F., SADOWSKY C., SAUNDERS R., REEVES A. (1977) *Alexia without agraphia, hemianopia, or color-naming defect: A disconnection syndrome.* Neurology 27: 689–691.

VRTUNSKI P., MACK J., BOLLER F., KIM Y. (1976) *Response to delayed auditory feedback in patients with hemispheric lesions.* Cortex 12: 395–404.

VRTUNSKI P., MARTINEZ M., BOLLER F. *The evaluation of delayed auditory feedback (DAF) effect: Comparison between subjective judgments and objective measures.* Cortex (in press).

WALTZ A. (1961) *Dyspraxias of gaze.* Archives of Neurology and Psychiatry 5: 638–647.

WARRINGTON E., JAMES M., KINSBOURNE M. (1966) *Drawing disability in relation to laterality of lesion.* Brain 89: 53–82.

WARRINGTON E., ZANGWILL O. (1957) *A study of dyslexia.* Journal of Neurology, Neurosurgery and Psychiatry 20: 208–215.

WEINSTEIN S. (1959) *Experimental analysis of an attempt to improve speech in cases of expressive aphasia.* Neurology 9: 632–635, 1959.

WEISENBURG T., McBRIDE K. (1935) *Aphasia. A clinical and psychological study.* New York, The Commonwealth Fund.

193

WERNICKE C. (1874) *Der aphasische Symptomenkomplex.* Breslau, Cohn und Weigert.

WERNICKE C. (1903) *Ein Fall von isolierter Agraphie.* Monatsschrift für Psychiatrie und Neurologie 13: 241–265.

WINGFIELD A. (1975) *Acoustic redundancy and the perception of time-compressed speech.* Journal of Speech and Hearing Research 18: 96–104.

WINGFIELD A., KLEIN J. (1971) *Syntactic structure and acoustic pattern in speech perception.* Perception & Psychophysics: 9: 23–25.

YAMADORI A. (1975) *Ideogram reading in alexia.* Brain 98: 231–238.

YATES A. (1963) *Delayed auditory feedback.* Psychological Bulletin 60: 213–232.

ZANGWILL O. (1960) *Le problème de l'apraxie idéatoire.* Revue Neurologique 102: 595–603.

ZANGWILL O. (1960) *Cerebral dominance and its relations to psychological function.* Edinburgh, Oliver and Boyd.

ZANGWILL O. (1967) *Speech and the minor hemisphere.* Acta Neurologica et Psychiatrica Belgica 67: 1013–1020.

ZANGWILL O. (1969) *Intellectual status in aphasia.* In VINKEN P., BRUYN G. (eds.) *Handbook of clinical neurology* IV. Amsterdam, North-Holland Publishing Company: 105–111.

ZURIF E. (1974) *Auditory lateralization: Prosodic and syntactic factors.* Brain and Language, 1: 391–404.

ZURIF E., MENDELSOHN M. (1972) *Hemispheric specialization for the perception of speech sounds: The influence of intonation and structure.* Perception and Psychophysics 11: 329–332.

ZURIF E., SAIT P. (1970) *The role of syntax in dichotic listening.* Neuropsychologia 8: 239–244.

ZUTT J. (1932) *Rechts-Linksstörung, konstruktive Apraxie und reine Agraphie.* Monatsschrift für Psychiatrie und Neurologie 82: 253–305, 355–395.

INDEX

195

197

JOURNAL OF CLINICAL NEUROPSYCHOLOGY

Editors:

Louis Costa   Byron P. Rourke

AIMS and SCOPE

The Journal of Clinical Neuropsychology will publish original articles dealing with research and theory in the broad field of behavioral impairment associated with dysfunction at the level of the cerebral hemispheres. The following general topics fall within the areas considered appropriate for inclusion in the Journal:

(1) the etiology, description, course, and prognosis for the psychopathological accompaniments of various types of brain disease;

(2) the development, reliability, validity, and utility of techniques of psychological assessment and intervention for persons suffering from brain impairment. Articles dealing with the delivery of service, case histories, experimental studies, epidemiological investigations, descriptive studies of patient groups, and theoretical articles are considered to fall within the purview of the Journal. Book reviews and reviews of research on subjects of fairly general concern will be solicited by the Editors. Examples of patient groups of interest would include adults with well-documented cerebral lesions, children with developmental dyslexia or some other form of serious learning abnormality, persons suffering from untoward psychological sequelae following head injury, etc. Each article should constitute an original contribution to knowledge concerning the topics outlined above.

To be ordered from
Swets PUBLISHING SERVICE
a division of Swets & Zeitlinger
347b Heereweg
2161 CA LISSE, Holland

SWETS NORTH AMERICA, INC.
P.O.Box 517
BERWYN, PA 19312, USA.

NEUROLINGUISTICS

Already published:

1) Y. Lebrun et al., THE ARTIFICIAL LARYNX.
   1973. 90 pp., 68 figs.   ISBN 90 265 0173 0   Dfl.   27.50

2) Y. Lebrun and R. Hoops, INTELLIGENCE AND APHASIA.
   1974. 140 pp., 3 figs.   ISBN 90 265 0182 X   Dfl.   27.50

3) H.W. Buckingham and A. Kertesz, NEOLOGISTIC JARGON APHASIA.
   1976. 100 pp.   ISBN 90 265 0227 3   Dfl.   37.50

4) Y. Lebrun and R. Hoops (Eds.), et al., RECOVERY IN APHASICS.
   1976. 270 pp., 31 figs.   ISBN 90 265 0228 1   Dfl.   62.50

5) W. von Raffler-Engel and Y. Lebrun (Eds.), et al., BABY TALK AND
   INFANT SPEECH.
   1976. 362 pp., 41 figs.   ISBN 90 265 0229 X   Dfl.   80.00

6) A.R. Luria, NEUROPSYCHOLOGICAL STUDIES IN APHASIA.
   1977. 184 pp., 6 figs., frontispiece
                            ISBN 90 265 0244 3   Dfl.   45.00

7) W. Riese, SELECTED PAPERS ON THE HISTORY OF APHASIA.
   1977. 144 pp., frontispiece
                            ISBN 90 265 0265 6   Dfl.   48.00

8) Y. Lebrun and R. Hoops (Eds.), THE MANAGEMENT OF APHASIA.
   1978. 124 pp., 3 figs.   ISBN 90 265 0280 X   Dfl.   45.00

Available through any bookseller or directly from the Publisher:

Swets Publishing Service, 347b, Heereweg, 2161-CA LISSE, Holland
Swets North America Inc., P.O. Box 517, BERWYN, PA 19312, USA